"Ventilator Man..."

Copyright © 2015 - 20...

**Copyright not claimed on reference pictures.
No part of this book may be reproduced in any manner, print, or electronic, without written permission of the copyright holder.**

The views expressed herein are those of the authors and do not necessarily reflect the views of your employer, medical director or current protocols.

This publication is intended to provide accurate information regarding the subject matter addressed herein. However, it is published with the understanding that FlightBridgeED, LLC is not authorizing or advising you to engage in unsafe practice or render care above your current state or county protocols. The information contained herein is solely for advanced education for licensed professionals wishing to further their knowledge base. It is not intended for the layperson to provide medical care. It should not supersede each individual's scope of practice or current medical policies and procedures for which the individual is covered under. It is the individuals' responsibility to use their own clinical judgment for decision-making and provide care in a manner consistent with current standards of care. The information in this publication is subject to change at any time without notice based on new research or treatment approaches that are standard in the medical industry. Neither FlightBridgeED, LLC nor the authors of the publication, make any guarantees or warranties concerning the information contained herein. If expert assistance is required, please seek the services of an experienced, competent professional in the relevant field. Accurate indications, adverse reactions, and dosage schedules for drugs may be provided in this text, but it is possible that they may change. Readers are urged to review current package indications and usage guidelines and protocols provided by the manufacturers of the agents mentioned.

Third Edition Printing – August 2018
FlightBridgeED, LLC
Headquarters
520 Old River Road
Scottsville, KY 42164
www.flightbridgeed.com

Contributing Editors

Ashley Bauer, MSN, MBA, APRN, NP-C, CFRN
President – FlightBridgeED, LLC
Editor in Chief
FlightBridgeED, LLC
Scottsville, KY 42164

Mike Herman, BSN, RN, CFRN
Flight Nurse
Enloe FlightCare
Chico, CA 95926

Evan Claunch, AAS, FP-C, CCEMT-P
Clinical Base Educator | Flight Paramedic
Air Methods Corporation
Systems Administrator | Web Developer
FlightBridgeED, LLC
Russell Springs, KY

Scott M. Gordon, BSN, RN, CFRN
Regional Clinical Compliance Evaluator
Air Methods Corporation – Mercy Air
Rialto, CA

FlightBridgeED, LLC
"Ventilator Management" – A Pre-Hospital Perspective

TABLE OF CONTENTS

CHAPTER   PAGE

DISCLOSURE..i
CONTRIBUTING EDITORS..ii
DEDICATION..iv
FOREWORD...v
PREFACE...vii
CHAPTERS
    CHAPTER 1 – Respiratory Physiology....................1
    CHAPTER 2 – Ventilator Terminology..................26
    CHAPTER 3 – Basic modes of Ventilation............76
    CHAPTER 4 – Advanced modes – Concepts..........97
    CHAPTER 5 – Ventilator Strategy........................111
    CHAPTER 6 – Alarms..124
    CHAPTER 7 – Pain and Sedation Management..126
    CHAPTER 8 – Case Application Commentary.....137
REFERENCE CHARTS..151
ABOUT US..154
REFERENCES..155

Dedication

To my amazing wife! You are my rock and my true love. Thank you for being that constant light that shines in my life. You've always been my biggest supporter and have given me so many gifts. We have an amazing love and I'll always be grateful for you and our life together. Thank you for loving me and being the woman you are! As I've said many times, you don't get enough credit for all you do with FlightBridgeED. Thank you for being that glue that holds things together. You are instrumental to the success of FlightBridgeED and this book! Thank you honey! Timing is everything!

Foreword

I have spent the last quarter century of my medical career in emergency departments and helicopters. During this time I have come to realize that if there is one skill that defines the specialty of critical care transport, it is airway management. But remember, airway management is not a single procedure such as endotracheal intubation or LMA placement. It's a spectrum of procedures, starting with basic airway maneuvers on one end, and surgical airways on the other. There are countless texts and journal articles available addressing airway management in the pre-hospital environment.

What seems to be too often glossed over is how to manage these critical patients after the airway is secured. Two decades ago, it was considered appropriate to transport most intubated patients using a BVM. This is certainly no longer the standard. All critical care transfers must be mechanically ventilated. Keep in mind that ventilator management involves so much more than dialing in a tidal volume, O_2 concentration and respiratory rate. In addition, all such patients must be treated with appropriate sedation and analgesia (Hint, it is not 5mg of Midazolam and 10mg of Vecuronium). Proper post-intubation care can have a profound effect on your patient's overall and neurologic survival. It is a skill that must be mastered by all medical personnel in the critical care transport field.

If you are in the business of transporting critical care patients, you MUST have a solid working knowledge of respiratory physiology, ventilator management and pharmacology. This cannot be taught in a 3-week or 3-

month paramedic/RN critical care course. It will require on the job education, frequent exposure to ventilated patients as well as an organized self-study program. This book is an excellent start and reference tool. Eric has done a wonderful job of condensing these incredibly broad subjects into a concise readable format. The contents of this text will provide any pre-hospital practitioner with a solid foundation as to the care of their critically ill ventilated patients.

Another excellent source of up to date pre-hospital critical care education, are the courses and podcasts offered by FlightBridgeED (the same people who wrote this book). Always remember, if you desire the best possible care for your patients, your initial certification and degree is just the first step of your life long educational journey.

Good luck!

Michael Abernethy, MD, FAAEM
Chief Flight Physician - UW Health Med Flight
Clinical Associate Professor of Emergency Medicine
University of Wisconsin School of Medicine and Public Health

Preface

Throughout the past 16 years working in the HEMS industry there have been many strides made industry wide to overcome the knowledge gap as it relates to mechanical ventilation. During my career as a flight paramedic and educator, I have gained a passion for furthering my knowledge and providing this essential education to medical crewmembers seeking to understand this important subject. Ventilator management is complex and causes a great deal of confusion among HEMS crews. Respiratory therapists receive extensive training on this subject. In contrast, flight nurses and flight paramedics are expected to gain competency through a crash course on this subject and then treat and stabilize various patient clinical conditions, with very little training in comparison to the two-four years of education respiratory therapists receive. It is often left up to the clinician to seek out other means of education so as to gain a more in-depth understanding.

The goal of this book is to provide the most up to date information based on current research and my experiences as a flight paramedic and educator. *"Ventilator Management" A Pre-Hospital Perspective*, will take a comprehensive look at ventilator management strategies as it relates to pre-hospital transport in both EMS and HEMS industries. The book is written in a comprehensive but conversational format and will hit on all things related to critical care transport ventilation. The book includes current research concepts, ventilation theory, core clinical ventilation strategies, and case application commentary, with reference materials for maximizing your study time.

Chapter 1 – Respiratory Physiology

Oxygenation and Diffusion

We have all learned, at some point in our educational career, whether in 7th grade biology class or during our college years, the definition of diffusion. Remember, diffusion is the process of a liquid or gas moving from a level of higher concentration to a level of lower concentration; equilibrium per se. We are always taught to provide high concentrations of oxygenation or FiO_2. But what does that mean, and how does that really work? There are multiple factors that affect gas exchange, including partial pressure of oxygen and cellular uptake. In this section, we will explore how oxygenation takes place and look at how diffusion facilitates that process.

When we think about oxygenation, it is important to understand the starting aspects of how much oxygen we breathe in and the effects on partial pressure (concentration). If you were sitting at sea level, the atmospheric pressure would be 760 torr (mmHg). Atmospheric oxygen concentration is always 0.21 or 21%. So, we need to understand how to calculate our partial pressure of oxygen prior to ever inhaling or bringing air into our oropharynx. We do this by multiplying atmospheric pressure (760 torr) at sea level, by the concentration of oxygen (.21). **Note:** (*If you see Atmospheric pressure in "torr" or mmHg they are considered the same unit of measurement essentially.*)

760 torr x .21 = 159.6

This is our starting partial pressure or PO_2. As we bring air into our nasopharynx, the air is humidified and thus diluted. To understand why it is diluted, imagine placing the same amount of oxygen in two containers of water. One container has 100 mL and the second container has 150 mL. The container with 150 mL would be more diluted compared to the 100 mL container. This is based on the water vapor pressure that is found in our environment. It is a fixed amount and accounts for 47 mmHg. This is the same concept. Because of this dilution, we see that the partial pressure of oxygen decreases from 159 to 104 [Figure 1-1]. So this is essentially the starting point for what is called the oxygen cascade. Oxygen cascade relates to oxygen traveling down our bronchioles, into our alveolar sacs and into our bloodstream for cellular uptake. At the same time, deoxygenated blood is returning from the heart via the pulmonary artery waiting to pass by the alveolar capillary membrane to be oxygenated. At this point, the partial pressure of arterial blood is approximately 40 mmHg. We have set the stage for diffusion, going into the mouth, the partial pressure is 104 mmHg and coming out from the heart, the partial pressure is 40 mmHg.

Figure 1-1: Example of Dalton's Law and partial pressure:
After dilution via humidification

Altitude (ft.)	Atmospheric Pressure (mmHg)	Alveolar Partial Pressure (PAO_2)
Sea Level	760	104
10,000	523	67
20,000	349	40
30,000	226	21

So, how does gas exchange occur? Gas exchange occurs via the alveolar-capillary membrane. This process utilizes diffusion and the concept of gas moving from an area of high concentration to an area of low concentration. Let's attempt to make this easier to understand. When you think of the alveolar membrane, imagine it as a large glass window. If our glass windows at home are dirty or blocked, we could not see through them or would not have the necessary light to do our daily activities. All of us want our windows clean and free of dirt. The alveolar membrane is no different. Think of it as the gatekeeper for oxygenation. If it is covered or filled with fluid (such as with ARDS or pneumonia), damaged (as occurs with atelectasis), overstretched (with high P$_{plat}$) or not sufficiently inflated (poor inspiratory maneuvers or hypoventilation), there will be no gas exchange across the membrane. This causes poor diffusion and end cellular oxygenation. This is called V/Q mismatch and shunt.

During this process, oxygen molecules have multiple collisions with the alveolar membranes, diffusing across the alveolar membrane into the capillary beds. The process of diffusion happens passively from the alveolus to the pulmonary capillaries. It then dissolves into the plasma and attaches to the hemoglobin (Hgb). Approximately 2% of the oxygen is dissolved and carried via the plasma with the rest being carried and stored on hemoglobin. Hemoglobin concentration is important in this process as well. Let's look at a patient with a normal hemoglobin concentration of 15 g/dL. This patient would carry 1.34 mL of oxygen on each Hgb molecule. This translates to approximately 1000 mL of oxygen uptake per minute if your patient had a normal Hgb concentration (15 g/dL), a normal cardiac output (Q) (5 L/min), and a normal SaO_2 of 100%. This is called the CaO_2 (content of O_2 in the arteries). We can calculate this easily with the following two formulas:

$$CaO_2 = (1.34 \times Hgb \times SaO_2) + PaO_2 \times 0.003$$

$$Do_2 = CaO_2 \times Q$$

If you look at the CaO_2 formula, you can see that the later half [+ PaO_2 x 0.003] of the equation gives an end number that is very small (0.3 mL). This is a representation of how much oxygen is dissolved and carried in the plasma. Remember, that is only 2-3% of the total oxygen. So, for purposes of really looking at this equation and understanding the amount of oxygen content in the arteries, using the first part of the equation gives you a more realistic representation of how much oxygen is attached to the hemoglobin. See below for example:

$$CaO_2 = (1.34 \times Hgb \times SaO_2)$$

$$Do_2 = CaO_2 \times Q$$

As you can see from the second formula **($Do_2 = CaO_2 \times Q$)**, we need the CaO_2 for the determination of the Do_2. We also need the current Q. To get the Q, we would need to have a Swan-Ganz catheter with a thermistor port to obtain that measurement. From there, we would need to covert the Q to a cardiac index (CI) based on each patient's body surface area (BSA). Using the CI is more accurate because everyone has a different BSA. However, often in the critical care transport environment, we will not have access to, or the ability to check this during flight, so the only way to trend this based on the above formula is to use recent data given by the transferring facility. In the end, the two biggest factors that will affect O_2 delivery are the hemoglobin concentration and the Q respectively.

So how do we apply strategies to improve oxygenation? First, let's think back to the alveolar membrane. We need to always think back to how we can make the membrane more efficient so oxygen molecules will move easier through the membrane. We do this by making that "glass window" cleaner, larger, and thinner. If we provide a good inspiratory volume that does not over-distend the alveoli, we are providing more surface area for the oxygen molecules to diffuse through. As such, by increasing the surface area, we are also making the membrane thinner, allowing for oxygen molecules to diffuse through quicker and without impedance. If we had an alveolar membrane that had a "shunt", we would essentially be saying that the membrane is blocked by some pathologic problem.

Let's look at a few examples. In a normal healthy lung, the membrane is normally very thin. However, in COPD or asthma, the membrane gets thicker due to fibrosis or restrictive interstitial diseases. The fibrosis leads to thickening of the alveolar membrane thus causing a V/Q mismatch and shunt. Furthermore, if the patient were suffering from pulmonary edema secondary to cardiogenic shock and failure, the alveolar membrane would be blocked by fluid build up in the alveoli. By providing better inspiratory volumes [6-8 mL/kg], and applying good PEEP, we are providing more surface area around that fluid build up and maintaining that surface area with good, safe PEEP strategies. Remember, inspiratory maneuvers (volume or pressure) recruit alveoli. PEEP is essential for maintaining the recruitment and functional residual capacity (FRC). If this process is altered, or slowed, it causes hypoxia. If it continues, it leads to hypoxemia (anaerobic metabolism and lactic acidosis). As before, we can look at cellular uptake of oxygen by our previous (CaO_2) formula. As such, we can also look at cellular use, or demand of oxygen, called the Fick formula and the Oxygen Extraction ratio. This is calculated in the following way:

$$VO_2 \ (1.34 \times Hgb \times SvO_2) + PaO_2 \times 0.003$$

$$O_2ER = (Oxygen\ Extraction\ ratio)$$
$$O_2ER = (CaO_2 - SvO_2) / CaO_2$$

Normal O_2ER is 25%

Meaning that Hgb passing through lungs to be oxygenated are 75% saturated during homeostasis

As with the CaO_2 formula from the previous page, we can disregard the last portion of the formula **(+ PaO_2 x 0.003)**. It represents a fraction of cellular demand as reflected by the amount of oxygen utilized from the plasma stores. As you can see from the formula, we need to have a current SvO_2 for this equation to give us trends on cellular demand. To get an SvO_2, the patient would need to have a central venous or pulmonary artery catheter in place. Many smaller hospitals will not place central lines, making trending of the SvO_2 difficult. However, new research and level-1 teaching facilities are trending this in their ICU's to guide their resuscitation. It is a useful tool in trending oxygenation at the cellular level and a tool that allows us to see if the patient in an anaerobic state is improving or worsening.

In the end, there are many factors that account for, measure, and affect oxygenation. Some of these concepts are more advanced. However, we can always go back to BLS techniques and think about optimizing the alveolar membrane surface area to see positive changes in the patient's oxygenation status and clinical course.

Ventilation

The process of ventilation refers to the body's regulation and maintenance of CO_2. Our normal CO_2 range is 35-45 mmHg. Any failure of this mechanism results in a ventilation problem or failure. Ventilation and oxygenation are very different. Often, clinicians confuse these concepts and make ventilator changes that are incorrect based on the pathophysiology involved. A proper understanding of both is essential in the critical care transport environment. In this section, we will discuss CO_2 production, regulation, and the different disease processes that affect different patient populations. Finally, we will discuss ventilator strategies that will assist you in your patient care and improve the patient's clinical course.

Before we get started on the pathophysiology of CO_2 regulation (ventilation), let's look at an example of ventilation and compare it to oxygenation. Often, traumatic brain injuries lead to brain death. However, the heart and organs are functioning fine. Remember, the respiratory centers are located in the midbrain via the medulla oblongata. To determine if a patient is brain dead, the physician will do a brain death study. During the study, the neurologist will place the patient on CPAP and take an initial ABG to identify the $PaCO_2$ and PaO_2. During the study, they watch the SpO_2, which will always stay at 95-100%. However, after a determined period of time they will run another ABG and look at the PCO_2. If the PCO_2 is elevated, then brain death is confirmed and the respiratory centers are dead. However, the patient will still be oxygenating fine and will most often have a perfect PO_2. Oxygenation is happening via simple diffusion at the alveolar membrane, however, there is no regulation of CO_2. Remember, CO_2 diffuses at a rate 20x faster than O_2. That means it is 20x more soluble than O_2. This is an important concept to understand, because even in severely ill patients, CO_2 diffusion is not the cause of the ventilatory failure. The patient may be hypercapnic, but this is not a result of poor diffusion. It will be due to respiratory muscle fatigue and failure in the COPD or asthmatic patient more often than not.

I think it is important to understand how CO_2 production takes place and how our bodies regulate this second-by-second (carbonic acid buffering system) and minute-by-minute (respiratory buffering system). Remember, we have an abundance of H+ and HCO_3^- with each counterbalancing the other to maintain homeostasis.

What mechanisms produce CO_2? The answer is aerobic and anaerobic metabolism! That is right, both do! Let's look at the aerobic state first. Remember that the glucose molecules split into (2) pyruvate molecules. Those pyruvate molecules split off and produce acetyl-CoA and CO_2. Once the CO_2 is produced, there is an intracellular CO_2 gradient that causes a shift out of the cell and into the blood. Of the CO_2 that diffuses into the blood, 93% of that CO_2 binds with the Hgb. However, about 70% of the CO_2 bound to the Hgb binds with H_2O to form carbonic acid in the plasma. Once the carbonic acid is formed it is split into H+ and HCO_3^-. The HCO_3^- is dumped into the blood as free-floating HCO_3^- and the H+ is attached to the red blood cells. In the end, 70% of the original CO_2 diffuses off of the Hgb and into the plasma as HCO_3^-. As the blood enters the lungs, this process is reversed and the CO_2 remaining is exhaled using the respiratory buffering system to finalize the process. This happens via the carbonic acid and respiratory buffering system second-by-second and minute-by-minute.

Furthermore, in an anaerobic state, we produce excessive amounts of CO_2 because of the quick glycolysis/fermentation phase that takes place. The bi-product of this oxidation process is lactic acid, ethanol, and CO_2. This causes a decreased pH and associated metabolic acidosis in our sick patients that have been in a prolonged anaerobic state.

How do we identify our CO_2 status? Does $EtCO_2$ = $PaCO_2$? What mechanisms are in place to regulate CO_2? First, as stated above, we need to have an aerobic state for proper CO_2 production and regulation. Our cells need to make CO_2 in the right amounts. Second, we need to have blood flow to the lungs. If we do not have adequate blood flow to the lungs, we cannot blow off the excess CO_2. The next thing is proper diffusion. As I stated above, CO_2 diffuses at a rate 20x faster that O_2. That means its 20x more soluble than O_2. If you had a diffusion problem related to CO_2 regulation, you would be dealing with a shunt (maybe a large pulmonary emboli). The last thing that you need to take into consideration is the patient's minute ventilation. This is the easiest way to regulate our patient's CO_2. We can classify this easily by looking at a normal CO_2 range. As stated above, the normal range is 35-45 mmHg. If your patient has a $PaCO_2$ >45 mmHg, that would be classified as alveolar hypoventilation. If your patient has a $PaCO_2$ <35 mmHg, that would be classified as alveolar hyperventilation.

How does $EtCO_2$ relate to $PaCO_2$? Is there a correlation? Yes and no. One of the newest and most important tools in the pre-hospital world is $EtCO_2$ quantitative waveform monitoring. This tool has become an invaluable tool for our intubation attempts and continued monitoring of airway control. With that being said, $EtCO_2$ can tell us more and can be used as a tool to improve the patient's metabolic disorder. Remember from the above section, we said that the normal values for CO_2 are 35-45 mmHg. Often times, this is the only way to identify the patient's CO_2 status. So how can we use this tool to turn around a patient's poor metabolic disorder? Remember, CO_2 is an acid, and with more acid in our body, our pH drops; with pH being the driving force for our body's homeostasis. So, if we understand this simple concept, we can turn a patient's pH toward the right direction by remembering these three simple rules. First, for every change in CO_2 by 10 mmHg, you will have a corresponding change in pH by 0.08 in the opposite direction. Second, in a normal person, the $PaCO_2$ and $EtCO_2$ will be within 3-5 mmHg from each other. With that in mind, please understand that the $PaCO_2$ will always be the highest number. Unless you have an ABG, you will truly never know the $PaCO_2$. However, the $EtCO_2$ will never exceed the actual $PaCO_2$. Furthermore, this is how we can utilize our $EtCO_2$ in an attempt to affect change in our overall ventilation status. Third, attempt to figure out the patient's current $PaCO_2$ – $EtCO_2$ gradient. How do we do this? When you get report on your patient, attempt to either get a new ABG or find out what the most recent ABG showed. Then, place the patient on your $EtCO_2$ quantitative waveform capnography and trend those results. Example: If the ABG showed the patient's last $PaCO_2$ was 75 mmHg, and your $EtCO_2$ shows 66 mmHg, then the gradient is 9.

Now let's use our first rule from above. For every change in CO_2 by 10 mmHg, you will have a corresponding change in pH by 0.08 in the opposite direction. Let's say this same patient, with an $EtCO_2$ of 66 mmHg, has a pH of 7.10 and $PaCO_2$ of 75 mmHg. Use your $EtCO_2$ reading and the gradient we identified to bring that pH up to near normal levels, with a perfect pH being 7.40. If we wanted to bring that 7.10 pH up to 7.34, we would need to drop our $EtCO_2$ by 30 mmHg. Remember, for every 10 mmHg change in

CO_2, the pH will change 0.08 in the opposite direction. We started with an $EtCO_2$ of 66 mmHg. We can use this tool to bring down the patient's pH by increasing their minute ventilation. Our goal is to attempt to slowly decrease the $EtCO_2$ from 66 mmHg to 36 mmHg. By using this technique during transport, you can bring the starting pH from 7.10 up to a near normal range of 7.34. Obviously this is just an example and there are other factors that play into metabolic disorders, but using this simple technique will aid in correcting a poor pH and help improve the patient's clinical course or outcome.

To expand on the idea of obtaining the $PaCO_2$ – $EtCO_2$ gradient, we are discussing a normal gradient versus an abnormal gradient, which tells you the level of shunt present in that patient. We have to remember that CO_2 diffuses very rapidly, actually 20x faster than O_2. Based on this, if you have a shunt that is affecting CO_2 gas exchange, it could potentially be significant. Obviously we have to remember that perfusion and overall cardiac output plays a big role in CO_2 removal and what is measured on the quantitative $EtCO_2$ capnography. With that being said, any perfusion related issues would be identifiable with a substandard $EtCO_2$, not one in the 60's. To go back to the patient discussed above, if the $PaCO_2$ was 75 mmHg and the $EtCO_2$ was 66 mmHg, the gradient is 9. To think about this in easier terms, to achieve a target $PaCO_2$ of 40 mmHg, the $EtCO_2$ would need to be titrated to 31 mmHg because this patient had an initial gradient of 9. Based on this, if we expand further and take the ratios from above and had an identifiable pH of 7.10 and wanted to attempt to make this pH 7.34, we could titrate our $EtCO_2$ from 66 mmHg to 36 mmHg, which would give us the pH of 7.34; although not perfect is heading in the right direction. This is just a teaching demonstration and in patients in severe metabolic acidosis, just changing the $PaCO_2$ is not going to correct the pH. However, in an isolated respiratory acidosis patient, this technique may be beneficial.

Understanding ventilation, CO_2 production and regulation is essential in treating respiratory patients. Furthermore, utilizing simple tools, as in $EtCO_2$ quantitative capnography, can not only help you monitor endotracheal tube (ETT) placement, but can help you monitor cardiac output and assist in fixing your patient's metabolic disorder.

Oxyhemoglobin Dissociation Curve

The oxyhemoglobin dissociation curve can be confusing. As such, I have attempted to make analogies that will foster our memories to hold on to some of this information. This concept is a critical aspect of everything we do in critical care and overall oxygenation delivery. It has become one of my favorite topics and I find it very fascinating. Now let's look at some analogies.

Think of the oxyhemoglobin dissociation curve as a "Manual for Dating". In a healthy relationship you have a good date, really like that person, but don't mind dropping them off after an evening out because you know you will see them again. Hemoglobin picks up and drops off O_2 when needed (normal curve).

In another scenario, you pick up your date, but do not like

them, so you cannot wait to get the date over. You drop them off fast! In a Right shift, hemoglobin has less affinity for O_2. This means that the O_2 cannot attach and be stored before the hemoglobin dumps it off to the tissues. You have a resulting lower than normal SpO_2, but excellent tissue oxygenation (PaO_2). In this situation, think everything that is Raised leading to a Right shift. Raised acid, Raised CO_2, Raised temp, Raised 2,3-DPG and Raised PaO_2.

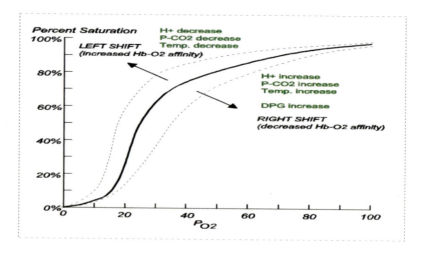

Why is this significant? Most of our patients will fall under this category. The raised acid levels are due to the increased CO_2 and H^+ ion levels. The potentially high 2,3-DPG can manifest from disease processes like COPD. These patients produce an increase in RBC. Because of the association of 2,3-DPG to RBC, you will have an increase in those molecules. Remember, the 2,3-DPG are the crowbars that "POP" off the O_2 molecules from the Hgb. It would make sense that the O_2 release seen in a right shift would be hyperdynamic in COPD patients, or for that matter any patient with increased levels of 2,3-DPG. Other people with potentially high levels may be athletes that train at high altitudes in an attempt to increase their RBC counts and people that live at higher altitudes on a daily basis. This is why people that live at, or train at high altitudes can readily use O_2 and have higher reserves.

In the end, patients suffering from a right shift on the oxyhemoglobin curve are going to have a lower than normal SpO_2 and higher than normal PaO_2. This will mean that they have higher than normal releases of O_2 stores to the tissues. It will also mean you will see lower SpO_2 readings. However, keep in mind that this does not mean your patients are hypoxic; your SpO_2 is only an indication of the Hgb saturation and nothing more. With that being said, right shift patients are not always getting oxygen molecules to the tissues either. Even though they have high PaO_2 levels, this does not mean that their shock state is allowing oxygen diffusion through to the tissues. Think about sepsis for example. If there is a diffusion shunt and interstitial fluid built up blocking access to the tissues, or access for diffusion through the alveolar-capillary membrane, your high PaO_2 means nothing. With that being said, if your Hgb releases its stores, then your SpO_2 will reflect lower, but as you can see, that does not represent the amount of O_2 being delivered to the tissues and organs.

In contrast, when considering a Left shift; you pick up your date, like them a lot, but you are insecure and do not want to drop them off. Jealousy!! Left shifts have higher affinity for O_2 and won't let the O_2 be dumped off to the tissues. This gives you a falsely high SpO_2, and poor tissue oxygenation (PaO_2). Remember, your SpO_2 is a reflection of the amount of O_2 bound to Hgb. If your Hgb is holding onto all the O_2 stores and not releasing them, you will have a highly saturated Hgb, but poor tissue oxygenation. Jealousy is BAD! In this situation, think everything Low; Low acid, Low temp, Low 2,3-DPG and Low PaO_2.

These patients are very sick. Basically, you will see this in metabolic alkalosis, hypothermia and massive transfusions of PRBCs. One of the biggest teaching points regarding the left shift is seen in trauma and massive transfusion guidelines. When looking at our treatment guidelines in trauma, we have learned that permissive hypotension is the key and that maintaining a MAP of 60-65 mmHg in a non-head injury patient will be sufficient to perfuse the brain and kidneys. In addition, massive transfusion protocols are now being employed. It is not uncommon to see patients receive 6-10 units of PRBCs in a 24-hour period. We have learned the most optimal is a 1:1:1 (FFP, platelets, PRBC) ratio as seen in the *PROPPR Randomized Clinical Trial*, by John Holcomb, M.D. et al., (2015). One of the biggest issues with massive transfusion, specifically regarding PRBCs is that the PRBCs are stored in citrate. The citrate kills off the 2,3-DPG molecules as well as binds with calcium found in the blood. Due to this, your patients are now bleeding out and having blood replacement that has a depleted amount of 2,3-DPG. Remember, this is an important molecule that helps release ("the crowbar") O_2 off the Hgb. Essentially, your patients will be moving from a right shift on the oxyhemoglobin dissociation curve to a left shift due to this phenomenon. It is important in these patients to fully resuscitate them with good oxygenation strategies and potentially even intubation and mechanical ventilation. Your SpO₂ may show normal or perfect, but that may be a false normal do to the left shift phenomenon and they actually may be having tissue hypoxia instead.

Graham's Law

Graham's law states that the rate of diffusion of a gas is inversely proportional to the square root of its molecular weight. This means that diffusion will happen at a faster rate if the gas is thinner and at a slower rate if the gas is heavier. First, let's discuss simple diffusion. We learned diffusion in our 7th grade science classes. Diffusion is the concept of a gas moving from an area of higher concentration to an area of lower concentration. We see this gas law in action when we breathe in atmospheric air and it is transported down to our alveolar sacs, where it moves across the alveolar-capillary membrane to the awaiting deoxygenated blood. The starting partial pressure of oxygen at the higher concentration moving into our alveolar sacs is 104 mmHg. Our partial pressure of oxygen in the deoxygenated blood returning from the heart is approximately 40 mmHg. This sets up the diffusion of oxygen moving from an area of higher concentration to an area of lower concentration. This not only happens at the alveolar level, but throughout the body in many facets.

Back to the aspect of diffusion as it relates to how heavy or thin the gas is. This is an important aspect of Graham's law. We see this when we look at the gases that make up atmospheric air. Atmospheric air is made up of 21% oxygen, 78% nitrogen, 1% hydrogen, argon, etc. The two gases that we will use to discuss this concept are oxygen and nitrogen. Oxygen is a thin gas and nitrogen is a heavy gas. When we bring in atmospheric air, it is primarily oxygen and nitrogen as stated above. The oxygen is essential for cellular function, as I have pointed out. This gas needs to diffuse very effectively and as such is thin and does just that. In contrast, nitrogen is a very dense, heavy gas that does not diffuse very well. It takes a lot to make it diffuse, and the only way to speed this up is by increasing the amount of oxygen concentration we provide for our patients. This aspect of nitrogen not diffusing very well is actually a good thing. Since nitrogen does not diffuse out of the alveoli very well, it is denser and acts like a cushion; it essentially acts as the prime ingredient in providing PEEP for our alveoli. Yes, PEEP! We need this gas to help provide adequate auto-peep in our lungs. We will discuss other aspects of nitrogen diffusion later in the FiO_2 section, but for purposes of Graham's law, I wanted to use this example to help illustrate the aspect of how diffusion is accomplished.

Henry's Law

Ok folks! Now let's talk about the most important gas law as it relates to oxygenation and ventilation. During my flight career, Henry's law has always been explained and taught to me in regards to decompression sickness and the basis of nitrogen being released into the joints and lungs. I never really understood the application as it related to my job. I guess if you live near the coast or in a community where diving is the big attraction, you may be able to put application into how this applies to your patient care. With that being said, I feel we have done a poor job representing this gas law. In this section we will look at Henry's law in a way that will allow you to really affect change in your patients. How? With oxygenation! Isn't that what counts most?

Before we get into how to apply this gas law, we first need to break down and define what it is.

Henry's law states the amount of gas dissolved in a solution is directly proportional to the pressure of the gas over the solution.

Ok, so what does that mean? How can this apply to oxygenation and ventilation? To be more specific, how does it apply to oxygen diffusion and CO_2 diffusion? Let's answer those questions!

One of the most important aspects of understanding ventilator management is how to apply changes to affect your patient is a positive way. Our goal is to be able to make changes based on oxygenation and ventilation, so your patient benefits from those changes, and their clinical course is improved. So how does it work?

Let's start with something we should all understand. What is the primary pre-treatment for our patients while being prepared for rapid sequence intubation? That's right: pre-oxygenation with high flow O_2. We do this by providing an increase in the FiO_2. This concept is the first aspect of applying Henry's law. We need to increase the concentration from an atmospheric oxygen of 21% to 100%. Imagine having a cup of water, with that cup of water representing the blood in our capillary beds that lie next to our alveoli. Then imagine putting in a handful of salt. That handful of salt represents atmospheric oxygen at 21%. All that salt is now floating around in the solution (blood). So if we apply Henry's law, now grab five handfuls of salt and add it to the cup of fluid. Now we have 100% oxygen and have increased the amount of oxygen molecules floating around in the blood. This causes the nitrogen to diffuse out of the alveoli because of the higher partial pressure of oxygen versus nitrogen. So, this concept is nothing new to you. The first thing we do when increasing oxygenation on ventilator patients is to increase FiO_2. A simple rationale for Henry's law is that if the partial pressure of a gas is twice as high than on average, twice as many molecules will hit the liquid surface in a given time interval, and on average twice as many will be captured and go into the solution.

Now let's examine the second rule of Henry's law. This is about increasing the surface area. Let's go back to that cup of water. Imagine that cup holds about 8 ounces and is 6 inches deep. If we were to pour that cup of water into a larger container, say a large mixing bowl, we would essentially be increasing the surface area available for oxygen molecules to diffuse through. So how do we accomplish this? By adding a safe amount of PEEP. That's right, by adding PEEP, you are maintaining alveolar recruitment and making the alveolar membrane, as well as the capillary beds, larger for oxygen molecules to diffuse through. It is that simple. When affecting change on our ventilator dependent patients as it relates to oxygenation, the first thing we do is increase the FiO_2 and the second step is to increase PEEP! Interestingly enough, they are the first two things in understanding Henry's law and applying it to your patient care.

Finally, lets look at the last step in applying Henry's law. We have increased the concentration as well as increased the surface area by applying PEEP. Now we need to put the solution (blood) under pressure. What does that mean? Well, by applying your ventilator, you are in-turn applying positive pressure by ventilating them by either volume or pressure ventilation. If you were to only have a BVM, ventilating them with good deep ventilations at the proper respiratory rate would apply enough pressure to pressurize the solution. Remember the statement from above:
A simple rationale for Henry's law is that if the partial pressure of a gas is twice as high than on average, twice as many molecules will hit the liquid surface in a given time interval, and on average twice as many will be captured and go into the solution.

Now we need to do something with all the increased oxygen molecules and the excellent surface area you created by your masterful PEEP application. By applying good volume or pressure-targeted ventilation, you will automatically apply enough pressure to push those oxygen molecules into the solution and help increase the amount diffused. This will translate to better O_2 pickup and cellular function down the line.

The understanding of this gas law is essential in how we respond to changes in our patient's condition. By utilizing this simple approach and by going back to the basics, you can really make a positive difference in your patients. In addition, you will become more confident in your management strategies and improve your patient's outcomes.

Dalton's Law

Dalton's law is essentially the law of partial pressure. Partial pressure is the pressure applied to a gas based on the barometric pressure it is put under. How does this apply to the HEMS industry? If you are flying rotor aircraft and staying below 2,500 feet, this gas law really is not that important for the everyday patient. It may play a role if you are flying a ductal dependent neonate, but that is a rare thing. If you are flying fixed wing, and flying at altitudes above 10,000 feet, then this gas law may have some relevance. So, let's look at this in more detail.

Dalton's law says that the total pressure of a gas mixture is the sum of the partial pressures of all gases. In addition, it describes how a pressure is exerted by a gas at various altitudes, and how that pressure affects the partial pressure of the said gas. So, how does that apply to our patients?

Remember, from the above section on oxygen diffusion, we said that at sea level our barometric pressure is 760 torr (mmHg). If we multiply (760 x 0.21 atmospheric oxygen) you get a partial pressure of oxygen of 159 mmHg. Let's apply this a little differently. Imagine you had a bag, and imagine having thousands of oxygen molecules floating around in that sealed bag. At sea level, they would be colliding with each other, and our body would be able to utilize them easily. Now, imagine you go up to 18,000 feet above sea level. At this altitude, the barometric pressure is 380 torr (mmHg). This is half of the pressure at sea level. If we take the same thought from above and multiply (380 x 0.21), this would give you a partial pressure of oxygen of 79 mmHg. Let's apply this the same way as above and look at the sealed bag of oxygen. We would still have the same concentration of oxygen in the bag, but because there is less pressure exerted against the bag, our oxygen molecules are floating around farther apart. There are far less collisions. This translates to less oxygen available for our body to pick up and utilize. Remember, everything that happens in our body is related to diffusion and partial pressure gradients. If our partial pressure is reduced, our ability to uptake and use oxygen efficiently becomes inadequate. This leads to hypoxia, and if prolonged, hypoxemia and cellular death.

As I stated in the beginning, Dalton's law is an important concept to understand, but really only applies to the flight crew that flies fixed wing, or does neonatal flights with infants that suffer from ductal lesions. However, by increasing the concentration, and applying the points laid out regarding Henry's law, you can overcome some of the problems associated with Dalton's law while flying at higher altitudes. If in doubt, always increase the concentration. You will be surprised at how many things this simple concept will correct.

A-a Gradient

The alveolar-arterial (A-a) oxygen concentration gradient is an important tool, and gives the clinician a really good insight of how the lungs and arterial system are communicating. Or better put, is there a ventilation/perfusion mismatch or shunt? It is a great identifying marker in the determination of the source of hypoxemia. This measurement helps isolate the location of the problem as either intrapulmonary (in the lungs) or extra-pulmonary (in the body).

A normal A-a gradient for a healthy young adult that is a non-smoker is in the range of 5-10 mmHg. Normally, the A-a gradient increases with age. A great calculation used to determine the gradient that occurs as we get older is as follows: **[(age in years)/4] + 4**. Thus, a 60-year-old adult non-smoker should have a physiologic A-a gradient of 19.

How do we apply this to our clinical picture and use it for understanding our patient's condition? The easiest way to apply this is to understand that an abnormally increased A-a gradient suggests a defect in diffusion. This is essentially the V/Q mismatch or right to left shunt we discussed earlier in this chapter.

As we are all aware, a low PO_2 indicates that the patient's current minute ventilation (whether high or low) is not enough to allow adequate oxygen diffusion into the blood. Therefore, the A-a gradient essentially demonstrates a high respiratory effort relative to the achieved level of oxygenation. That being said, a high A-a gradient could indicate a few things. It can show the patient is attempting to breathe hard to achieve oxygenation, the patient is breathing normally and attaining low oxygenation, or the patient is breathing hard and still failing to achieve normal oxygenation.

In contrast, if the lack of oxygen is due to a low minute ventilation, or respiratory effort (hypoventilation), then the A-a gradient is not increased. A healthy person who hypoventilates would have hypoxia, but a normal A-a gradient.

This is an easy concept to put into practice. As such, there are two ways to identify the A-a gradient. There is the old fashioned way. Yes, doing a little math. If interested, below is the calculation. In addition, there are many apps on the iPhone and Android devices that have A-a gradient calculators and will make using this useful calculation easy and quick at the same time.

$$Aa\ Gradient = \left(150 - \frac{5}{4}(P_{CO_2})\right) - P_aO_2$$

As you can see, this can be cumbersome while flying and may be difficult at night, and when you are dealing with a sick patient. That being said, just download a free app with the easy A-a gradient calculator and you are set. Furthermore, use this simple but effective calculation to help you identify why your patient is not oxygenating well. If you do so, you may be able to pinpoint the cause and fix the problem

Chapter 2 – Ventilator Terminology

Tidal Volume (V_t)

Tidal volume is the amount of volume delivered with each breath, and is measured and calculated in mL. Tidal volume has been a hot topic in recent years, with many studies conducted for the determination of how much V_t is appropriate. This has led to our understanding of ventilator lung injury (VLI), acute respiratory distress syndrome and the associated problems seen when high tidal volumes are delivered. Not too long ago, it was the norm to give patients V_t as high as 10-15 mL/kg. Often, we still see this in smaller hospitals where evidence based practice may not always be in place. As such, our patients may still be getting V_t as high as 800-1000 mL. What I have witnessed by many respiratory therapists in their V_t approach is to increase V_t as high as possible so as not to exceed a P$_{plat}$ of 30 mmHg. If that means a V_t as high at 1000 mL, then that is appropriate based on that practice. Why? They are attempting to recruit as many alveoli as possible without increasing alveolar pressures to unsafe levels. Again, I do not see the point and feel you can recruit alveoli in safer ways. In this section, we will discuss the new research and approach to V_t delivery and look at why this new approach is making a difference in our patient's clinical course and overall outcomes.

In recent years, a research group, called ARDS Network, has conducted many trials and published their findings on their website (http://www.ardsnet.org). This group of researchers has dedicated themselves to lowering the incidence of VLI and ARDS secondary to high V_t by conducting lower V_t trials. An example of one such trial is the ARMA study, which was a randomized, controlled multi-center 2 x 2 factorial study. It consisted of a drug treatment (ketoconazole vs. placebo) and a ventilation strategy (6 mL/kg tidal volume vs. 12 mL/kg tidal volume) to determine clinical outcomes. This study showed favorable clinical outcomes and a decreased incidence of VLI and ARDS while using the lower Vt strategy (ARDS Network, 1997). As such, we are now seeing and using the 4-6 mL/kg for all patients throughout the country, with a standard starting range of 6 mL/kg.

We have to realize that everything we do in medicine should mimic our physiologic norms. We breathe at a minute ventilation of 4-8 L/min. This translates to a V_t of 400-600 mL per breath. We don't need, nor do we utilize, anymore than that. So why give our patients a Vt higher than what we normally breath on a physiologic basis, which is 6 mL/kg? Remember, our alveoli are sensitive little sacs that are used for oxygenation processes. If we damage them, hyperinflate those sacs or cause atelectasis, we are defeating the purpose of optimizing our oxygenation and ventilation by using our ventilator as a tool for improving clinical course.

With all that being said, I feel starting at a V_t range of 6 mL/kg in most patients is optimal and will provide you with an appropriate V_t that is close to our patient's physiologic norm. By doing so, your patients will be more comfortable, will not need as much pain management and sedation and will have a lower incidence of VLI and ARDS. However, there may be patients that have large-healthy lungs that need higher volumes. Athletes and people with more physiologic lung volume may need starting V_t of 8 mL/kg. You will need to make this determination at the bedside. Additionally, patients with diseased lungs that have secondary enlargement or patients that have larger lung compliance may need higher starting V_t at 8 mL/kg. However, there has been countless studies showing that V_t ranges > 8 mL/kg cause ALI, whether those patients had healthy lungs or not. An excellent observational look at all literature published on this topic is a (June 2016) study by: **Davies et al., Should A Tidal Volume of 6 mL/kg be Used in All Patients?**

As I stated above, we need to protect our patient's lungs. Physiologic V_t is 6 mL/kg in most patients. By decreasing the V_t, it would make sense that we would need to increase the respiratory rate, so as to provide adequate minute ventilation. I will discuss this approach in more depth in later sections and bring this approach together with how to determine your minute ventilation as well as how to optimize oxygenation by adding proper amounts of PEEP.

Respiratory Rate (RR)

Your patient's respiratory rate (RR) is the other important component in determining their overall minute ventilation. Historically, we have seen patients with higher V_t and lower RR. This has changed as I have illustrated above. Now we have lower, more physiologic V_t, and higher RR in comparison to yesteryear.

In later sections, I will illustrate how minute ventilation is one of the most important concepts in overall oxygenation and ventilation. Understanding this concept will help you provide more efficient care to your ventilator dependent patients. As such, understanding that you need lower V_t as I have laid out and higher RR is important. Why? Again, we need to realize that doing everything as close to physiologic norms as possible will greatly benefit your patients. So how fast do most of us breath? I would argue between 16-18 breaths per minute. So why do I always see RR on our ventilator patients in the 8-12 range? This makes no sense; we don't breath this slow and surely need more while having some type of disease process, increased oxygenation demand or hypoxia.

Based on everything we have discussed in the above sections regarding V_t and overall minute ventilation, it is appropriate to start all your patients with a RR of 16-18 breaths/min. It will make more sense in the next section, but just remember this is a good physiologic norm and a range that will allow you to better meet or exceed your patient's metabolic oxygenation demand and minute ventilation needs without causing or starting the process of VLI. Remember, lower V_t and higher RR equal better patient comfort, and possibly clinical outcomes based on the trials I've quoted above. In addition, I will also show you two different approaches to applying protection with V_t and RR based on your patient's disease process. As such, the V_t and RR will change based on each approach.

Minute Ventilation (V_E)

Minute ventilation is one of the most important concepts and aspects of setting up your patient's ventilator settings and overall strategy. How to accomplish this in a manner that optimizes oxygenation and ventilation as well as protects your patient from the potential deadly combination of VLI and ARDS is essential. In this section, we will look at how to apply appropriate V_t and RR as well as look at how minute ventilation comes into play when discussing dead space and overall alveolar minute ventilation.

This concept is the teaching of **Dr. Scott Weingart** from the EMcrit podcast. Once I learned this simple concept and started applying this to my patients, I really saw a big difference in how my (V_E) maintained a proper $EtCO_2$. I then tweaked this formula based on conversations with Dr. Dan Davis. Let's examine this further! As I have stated a few times, we need to do everything in the most physiologic way possible while delivering our V_t and RR. Minute ventilation (V_E) can be defined as V_t x RR. So what is our physiologic norm when looking at V_E? While you are sitting here reading this delightful book, you are consuming approximately 60cc/kg/min of oxygen. This translates to the 4-8 L/min of minute ventilation we have always learned. So how does this calculation apply to your intubated, ventilated patients? When we intubate our patients, we increase what's called dead space. Dead space ventilation (V_D) can be defined as the amount of volume lost due to anatomic aspects, expansion of the ventilator circuit, ETT and any extensions added to the ventilator circuit, like an in-line suction catheter. As I stated above, we need to look at minute ventilation from two angles. First, overall V_E [the amount delivered based on V_t and (RR)] and alveolar minute ventilation (V_a) (the amount that reaches the alveolar level for gas exchange); with the latter being the most important. So how much dead space volume do we lose with each breath? We lose approximately 1mL/lb/IBW or an even easier number is 150 mL per breath. How do we account for this in a way that allows us to optimize alveolar minute ventilation? Simple! We take the 60 mL/kg/min we stated above and double it. That's right...double it! This is where I have tweaked this a bit. Dr. Scott Weingart taught 120mL/kg/min. However, after working with Dr. Dan Davis I have lowered this to 100mL/kg/min. This calculation will be your saving grace when managing your patients. As such, write this down or store it in you brain somewhere! This formula will allow you to provide an adequate V_E, while accounting for the loss in volume due to dead space and give you an adequate alveolar V_E. So let's do a few calculations below and look at why this formula works.

Let's say we have an 80 kg patient based on ideal body weight.

Formula: V_E = **100mL/kg/min**

V_E = 100mL x (80kg)= 8000mL or 8.0L/min

This is now the target V_E: **8000 mL**

Now we have to find out V_t.

The starting Vt is **4-6mL/kg**

The patient is **80kg x 6mL = Vt 480**

So the starting Vt is **480 mL**

Remember from above, your V_E is equal to your V_t x RR. Now we have the desired V_E (**8000 mL**) and V_t (**480 mL**). Now we just need to do a little division to determine the RR.

8000 / 480 = 16.6 breaths per minute. That's right **16.6** per minute. I tend to round down to 16. You can surely use 17 as well. What you will find is that in all situations, the RR will always come out between **16.6 (16)** while using **V_t of 6 mL/kg.**

Your end result is this:
Desired V_E = **8000 mL or 8.0 L/min**
Vt = **480 mL**
RR = **16**

As you can see, your desired and overall V_E is higher than the physiologic norms when it comes to minute ventilation as I lay out above (4-8 L/min). But remember, we lose up to 150 mL per breath in dead space (V_D). If we did this calculation to identify how much that is on this patient it would be:

RR (16) x 150mL (dead space) = 2400 mL or 2.4 L/min

If we subtracted this from our finished V$_E$ of 8.0 L/min, you would have an end result that would represent overall alveolar minute ventilation (V$_a$):

$$8.0 \text{ L/min} - 2.4 \text{ L/min} = 5.6 \text{ L/min } (V_E)$$

As you can see, this is right in the middle of our physiologic norm of 4-8 L/min. It allows for dead space and gives you, the clinician, the minute ventilation needed to meet metabolic demands and oxygen consumption on your sick, ventilator dependent patients.

Now let's look at a patient using the old way of just entering in a V$_t$ and RR and not accounting for dead space. Let's use the old V$_t$ of 500 mL and RR of 10 as our calculating numbers. I am positive you have seen many patients on these settings. I would also argue that you might have struggled to maintain the ventilation aspects, or needs, as it relates to eucapnia.

Calculation: (Vt) 500 mL x (RR) 10 = 5000 mL or 5.0 L/min

Now, let's subtract the dead space as we did in the above formula.

(RR) 10 x 150 mL (dead space) = 1500 mL or 1.5 L/min

If you take the dead space calculation of 1.5 L/min and subtract that from your V$_E$ of (5.0 L/min) you will get an end result of 3.5 L/min of V$_a$.

$$5.0 \text{ L/min} - 1.5 \text{ L/min} = 3.5 \text{ L/min}$$

$$V_a = 3.5 \text{ L/min}$$

This is at the bottom end of the physiologic norm we stated in the above sections and does not account for a patient's increased oxygen demand or hyperdynamic state often seen in our sick patients. Therefore, it is essential to understand the importance of how overall V_E and the end result of V_a impacts your patient's oxygenation and ventilation status. Like I said in the earlier part of this section, remember the 100 mL/kg/min formula and use it on all your ventilator patients.

Now that we understand V_E and V_a, let's take a look at a patient scenario that challenges many people in critical care medicine. I believe we can learn from this and apply some useful concepts at the same time. The below scenario will be the guiding scenario throughout this book. We will look upon it often and apply different concepts based on the chapter and section we are currently working in.

You and your partner respond in your BK-117 rotor aircraft to a small facility for a transfer of a 22-year-old female patient that has a diagnosis of possible DKA. Her current labs and ABGs indicate that she is suffering from severe metabolic acidosis. During your report, you are told that the patient is not intubated and breathing at a rate of 36 per minute. She has vomited x2 per the referring RN. You note that her SaO_2 is 88% on a NRB mask. You are told that your patient has a long history of IDDM and anorexia. The patient has been in this condition per family for approximately 48 hours prior to her arrival in the E.D. Upon assessment you and your partner decide that placing an advanced airway via RSI and ETT placement would benefit your patient. Your current ABG and labs are as follows:

pH 7.08, $PaCO_2$ 17, HCO_3^- 15, PaO_2 76

Labs: Na^+ 186, K^+ 2.2, Hct 68, Serum Osm 356, Glu 891, BUN 20, Cr 1.2

Currently on an insulin drip @ 11units/hr

She has (1) 18g IV in her left AC with a total of 500 mL of NS given prior to your arrival

No urine output via Foley

As you can tell, this patient scenario has many factors and aspects to consider while making your treatment decisions. In this section we are going to just look at her minute ventilation needs and the importance of understanding how that can either kill her, if managed wrong, or improve her clinical course if managed correctly.

When looking at this scenario and the ABG results, your first order of business is to identify if your patient is currently in a metabolic acidosis. If she is, it is important to make sure you maintain her current compensatory respiratory rate so as to not drop her pH any lower. We will look at that concept in more depth later in the book, but just know there is a correlation between your $PaCO_2$ and pH. If one goes up, the other drops in the opposite direction. So if your patient's $PaCO_2$ increases in this scenario, her pH will drop even more. It's already at a critical low of 7.08. So how do we deal with this? We deal with it just like we would with anyone suffering from a metabolic acidosis. How are they compensating? They are attempting to blow off as much acid (CO_2) as possible by increasing their respiratory rate. That is what causes the Kussmaul respirations we see in many metabolic acidosis presentations. By doing so, they are assisting in the compensation aspect of the respiratory buffering system and keeping the acid from building up even more, thus causing a decrease in the pH. You have one of the best tools available to you for every patient: your $EtCO_2$ quantitative waveform capnography. This will give you a starting guide in maintaining your patient's current compensatory status. If she is running at 15 on her $EtCO_2$, then that is where you need to maintain her once you intubate and establish your advanced airway. It is also essential to make sure you get the airway as quickly as possible. The most experienced provider needs to be handling the intubation.

Once you have your patient intubated and you begin your ventilator set up, you can use another easy calculation that will remind you of the need for the higher RR so as to maintain the compensatory rate and not drop the pH further. If you remember from above, our standard intubated V_E formula is 100 mL/kg/min. Based on that we said that in most calculations the RR will end up at 16. Ok...so if we use that as a starting point and realize we are needing a formula that represents a V_E in a metabolic acidosis patient, then we will use the following formula: **240mL/kg/min.** If you notice, this is more than double our normal intubated patient's desired V_E. By using the **240mL/kg/min**, you will have a RR in the range of 36-40/min. This will allow for continued compensation and protect the pH from decreasing further. If we didn't use the larger formula, and didn't increase the RR, you would cause the patient's CO_2 to increase, thus causing your patient to have a precipitous drop in pH and possible death. Again, we will look at the pH and $PaCO_2$ correlation later in the book, but just know that for every increase in $PaCO_2$ of 10 mmHg, you will have a corresponding drop in pH of 0.08. You can see that any increase in $PaCO_2$ can cause a quick drop in the pH.

Therefore, the teaching point to this scenario as it relates to V_E is to maintain a high V_E to protect the pH. By forgetting this important concept, you will most likely worsen your patient's clinical course and possibly cause the patient's death by mismanaging this simple, but important concept.

In this section, we will look at how the patient's exhaled tidal volume will give you the best indication of volume received by the patient. Essentially, it gives you an actual breath to breath glimpse of the variations seen with how the patient's lung compliance is affecting overall minute ventilation.

The exhaled tidal volume (V_{te}) is a parameter that you monitor on any ventilator's settings screen and gives you a second-by-second account of chest wall compliance and volume delivered compared to volume received. Most literature will tell you that you should see a +/- 50 mL variation from your V_t and your V_{te}. With that being said, don't get too caught up on that number. There are however a few things to consider. Always confirm you have good chest compliance and the difference is not a result of impending poor compliance. With that being said, each ventilator circuit has compliance loss in volume. For an adult circuit (any patient > 20 kg) it is (1.4mL x PIP), and round it up to (2mL x PIP). In contrast, for pediatric circuits (pediatrics circuits are used for any pediatric < 20kg), it is (0.8mL x PIP). Again round it up to (1mL x PIP) and add that to your calculated Vt. Example: Your V_t: 400, V_{te}: 360, PIP 20 cmH$_2$O. Your compliance loss based on the circuit is (2mL x 20) = 40mL. You then add this to your V_t and you account for the loss seen in the circuit. Your V_t would now be set at 440 mL to account for this difference. This is the only time you would just increase your V_t based on a lower V_{te}. Again, any other time always confirm you don't have a compliance issue, air-trapping or impending pneumothorax.

When we look at V_{te} as a tool for lung compliance status, it is important to note any variation and look at the pathophysiology related to the patient's disease process. If the patient is a COPD patient and has poor chest wall compliance or has been suffering from breath stacking or auto-PEEP and you see the V_{te} variation start to decrease, then you need to understand it is an indication of the patient's chest wall compliance diminishing.

Example: You have a patient you are providing a V_t of 500 mL and your V_{te} has been running 420 mL. Then over 5 minutes, you notice that your Vte has decreased from the 420 mL to 230 mL. This should immediately raise your internal alarms! This is a bad sign and a problem that needs correcting quickly. If it is secondary to a COPD patient that is breath stacking and has increased auto-PEEP, then removing them from the ventilator for a 30 second period and allowing them to exhale all that stored volume will correct the problem. This is essentially reducing the auto-PEEP phenomenon. In contrast, if you see this phenomenon in a trauma patient and note based on your initial assessment that the patient had a potential for a pneumothorax, then correcting this problem with chest decompression is warranted and will be needed immediately. This is a life threatening situation and one that needs to be taken seriously!

We will look at the V_{te} a bit closer when we dive into the different aspects of pressure control ventilation (PCV), but at this point I will leave it at that. Understanding this important but easy to use tool is essential and will give you a great glimpse of how your patient's lung compliance is changing for the better or worse.

I:E Ratio

In this section, we will define and discuss the use and meaning of I:E ratio and how this important tool is utilized to affect change for your patient's ventilation and oxygenation status. When looking at the I:E ratio and defining its use, often it is only looked at and used for affecting your patients ventilation status. In simpler terms it is used to affect change with regards to your patient's CO_2 regulation or exhalation time. I would argue that dealing with your patient's exhalation time is one of the most challenging aspects of ventilator management. The first phase of the I:E ratio is your inhalation time. Your inhalation time is always active; therefore it requires less time than expiration and is an easier process to complete. We tend to not think about breathing in. In contrast, your exhalation is a passive process that requires more time for the alveolar units to empty. As such, if the expiratory time is of insufficient duration, your patient will suffer gas trapping, which will lead to what is called "auto-PEEP".

I:E ratio, or inspiratory:expiratory ratio, refers to the ratio of inspiratory time vs. expiratory time. In normal spontaneous breathing, the expiratory time is most often twice as long as the inspiratory time. This gives an I:E ratio of 1:2, which is standard for most adult patients. However, this ratio is typically changed in COPD and asthmatics, or obstructive lung patients, due to the prolonged time needed for expiration. They might have an I:E ratio of 1:3 or 1:4. Even longer expiratory times are required at times, but this is best done after gaining a broader understanding of this process. Below is an example of how a standard I:E ratio of 1:2 looks based on the inspiratory:expiratory time:

Your patient has a RR set at 10

You divide 60 sec by 10 (breaths per minute)

60/10 = 6 sec respiratory cycle

If your I:E ratio was set at 1:2 you would have to divide this by the 6 sec respiratory cycle

That would mean your inspiratory time = 2 sec and your expiratory time = 4 sec

As you can see, your expiratory time is longer by 2 sec in the above example.

There are times when an experienced clinician can use the I:E ratio to affect positive change with regards to oxygenation. This is accomplished by inversing the I:E ratio. Inversing the I:E ratio allows for a longer inhalation phase and shorter exhalation phase. Why? Remember, when delivering volume, your goal is to recruit as many alveoli as possible without causing VLI or excessive pressures. So by inversing the I:E ratio, you are in turn prolonging the inhalation phase and causing better alveolar recruitment, preventing atelectasis and providing a better surface area for oxygenation. Only very experienced clinicians should attempt this technique and it is most often only found in protocols with guidance by medical direction. Furthermore, applying inverse I:E ratios (3:1, 4:1) can only be done in pressure control ventilation (PCV), not in a volume mode. Understanding this important concept and tool to improve the clinical course of your patient with severe hypoxemia or non-compliant lungs could make the difference between survival and death.

I-Time

Inspiratory time is a reflection of the overall I:E ratio and changes based on a change to the I:E ratio. Inspiratory time is the time over which the tidal volume is delivered (volume delivery) or the pressure is maintained (pressure delivery) depending on the mode of delivery. I often get asked this question: What is the difference in I-time and rise-time? Think of it this way. If delivering a breath with pressure control ventilation, imagine you are going on vacation to Disney World. Your rise-time is the time is takes to get to Disney World and your I-time is the amount of time you stay at Disney World. In the time cycled modes, either inspiratory time or I:E ratio is set and adjusted to ensure that the set Vt is delivered in that time. Examples of these modes are pressure control ventilation (PCV) and pressure regulated volume control (PRVC). In contrast, during volume control cycled modes, the I-time is set and inspiration ends when the set Vt is reached. Most often, using your I:E ratio to adjust for your inhalation vs. exhalation time is the easiest and most efficient way to do so.

If this is confusing, I would always refer to your I:E ratio as a guide to your inhalation and exhalation understanding and manipulation. Remember, by adjusting your RR and I:E ratio, you are in turn affecting your I-time. Refer to figure 2-1 on next page for a sample of how I-time relates to I:E ratio.

There is one circumstance where the clinician will use the I-time instead of an I:E ratio to adjust inhalation vs.

exhalation time. When providing time cycled ventilations (PCV or PRVC) on a neonate or little pediatric patient, the clinician needs to use an I-time of 0.3-0.5 seconds to be able to get the Vt delivered at an I:E ratio of 1:1 with associated low tidal volumes. What I mean by this setting is that when using small Vt and attempting to deliver an I:E ratio of 1:1 that is most often required on neonates, one has to use the I-time to deliver that ratio.

(f)	**(I-Time)**	**(I:E Ratio)**
10	2.0	1:2
12	1.5	1:2.3
15	1.3	1:2.1
20	1.0	1:2.0
25	0.8	1:2.0
30	0.6	1:2.3
40	0.5	1:2.0

Figure 2-1: Example of RR vs. I-time vs. I:E ratio chart for an I:E ratio of 1:2

Flow

Flow is something that most of us don't really understand with regards to our ventilator patients. Why? One big reason is that our transport ventilators, although excellent, do not have an option to adjust flow, as you would see in a high level ICU ventilator. Essentially what you have on the LTV1000, 1200 or ReVel ventilators is something called Vcalc. This is essentially the flow that is based on the overall minute ventilation and I-time. Although we cannot truly change this, we can understand it and know how to calculate it.

$$\text{Flow} = 60\text{L/min} \quad V_t = 500 \text{ mL} \quad \text{I-time} = 1 \text{ sec}$$

$$\frac{60\text{L}}{\text{min}} = \frac{1\text{L}}{\text{sec}} = \frac{1000\text{mL}}{\text{sec}}$$

$$\frac{1 \text{ sec}}{1000\text{mL}} \times \frac{500\text{mL}}{x} = \frac{500}{1000} = 5/10 = 0.5 \text{ sec}$$

As you can see from the above formula, the ventilator told us that we were delivering 60 L/min of flow. We have to use good old-fashioned algebra to reduce this down and identify what that equals per second. As you can see, I have reduced 60 L/min down to 1000 mL/sec and cross-canceled to get an answer of 0.5 sec. What that means is that 60 L/min of flow is delivering a V_t of 500mL over 0.5 sec. As you can imagine, being able to alter this can really affect your patients. Being able to deliver a breath over 1 sec instead would increase alveolar recruitment and affect oxygenation potential in a positive manner.

One tool the LTV1000, 1200 and ReVel ventilators have when in PCV that can help you alter the length of delivery, or "slope", is to go into the back settings menu and change the "rise time" profile. These ventilators have nine different rise time profiles that change the slope of delivery (how long the inspiratory slope is held) by 33% with each profile from 1-9. The ventilators will default to a rise time profile of (4). I would recommend trying this and playing with a test lung to visually see the difference when using the different profiles, with a profile of (1) delivering the breath fast and a profile of (9) delivering the breath over a longer period.

Fraction of Inspired Oxygen (FiO$_2$)

Oxygen is something we all understand and have been taught to administer when in doubt. It is the one medication that we can give to most of our patients and see a positive change. But how does oxygen, or I should say FiO$_2$, affect our ventilator patients? How do we administer it? As we explained in the gas laws section, the first and most important gas law is Henry's law. As such, when applying Henry's law, we said that our first action was to increase the concentration. We do this by increasing the FiO$_2$, which will improve oxygenation in all situations. With that being said, there are a few things we need to understand about oxygen.

Oxygen is a true biological toxin and our body does not need high amounts; we live just fine on 0.21 or 21%. So what happens when we have high concentrations of oxygen for long periods of time? Let's take a look at the pathophysiology involved. If we remember from the first section on aerobic metabolism, normal cellular respiration involves the addition of four single electrons to the O_2 molecule (conversion of O_2 to H_2O). During normal partial pressure (104 mmHg), 95% of the molecules will be reduced to H_2O and 5% will be partially reduced to toxic metabolites or what are called free radicals (FR). The FRs then leak into the cytosol, and out from the cell. FRs attack the lipids, proteins, and nucleic acids of the cells and tissues. This in turn causes decreased protein synthesis and is very hard on lung tissue and cells and causes increased mucus production and the start of a huge inflammatory cascade that can lead to ARDS and DIC in severe cases.

Absorptive Atelectasis

Another important concept to understand about prolonged use of high FiO_2 is the concept of absorptive atelectasis. Absorptive atelectasis is an important aspect of oxygen toxicity that results from 100% FiO_2 displacing all the nitrogen that normally sits in the alveoli acting as the PEEP. It instead pushes it out of the alveoli, causing alveolar collapse.

Let's take a closer look at this phenomenon. Oxygen shares alveolar space with other gases, principally nitrogen. Nitrogen is poorly soluble in plasma, and thus remains in high concentrations in alveolar gas. If the proximal airways are obstructed, for example by mucus plugs, the gases in the alveoli gradually empty into the blood along the concentration gradient, and are not replenished. Therefore, the alveoli collapse by a process known as atelectasis. This is limited by the sluggish diffusion of nitrogen. If nitrogen is replaced by another gas, that is if it is actively "washed out" of the lung by either breathing high concentrations of oxygen, or combining oxygen with more soluble nitrous oxide in anesthesia, the process of absorptive atelectasis is accelerated. It is important to realize that alveoli in dependent regions, with low V/Q ratios, are particularly vulnerable to collapse. Ok, so let's break it down based on our previous sections. When we breathe in atmospheric air, remember it is made up of 21% oxygen and 78% nitrogen along with other gases that are not relevant to this discussion. Nitrogen is a very dense/heavy gas; a gas that is very sluggish with regards to diffusion. As such, when we bring in atmospheric air, the oxygen in that air diffuses through the alveolar membrane and attaches to the Hgb and dissolves in the plasma. The 78% nitrogen just hangs out and stays in the alveoli. Therefore, it does not diffuse well and acts as a pillow or PEEP for the alveoli and essentially keeps the alveoli from collapsing. We need this! This is important! If we did not have this gas, our alveoli would collapse, thus causing atelectasis and alveolar trauma.

If you remember, we essentially do this everyday while performing RSI. We are taught to give high concentrations of FiO_2 in the attempt to raise our patients PO_2 and cause nitrogen washout. However, if we were to give 100% FiO_2 for long periods (days), we would see the high concentrations of oxygen start displacing the nitrogen. The oxygen would then occupy the entire alveolar space and once the O_2 diffuses into the capillary beds, there would be no nitrogen left in the alveoli, thus causing alveolar collapse.

So how much is too much and when is too much a bad thing? We should always give the highest amount of oxygen in the hopes to raise our patients PO_2 back to normal levels. In addition, FiO_2 in the trauma and pregnancy population is essential and important. Remember, we need to do whatever possible to optimize oxygenation with any patient population. In the trauma patient, we are trying to overcome hypemic hypoxia, as our oxygen carrying capacity is most likely decreased. If we have deficient Hgb levels, we will have poor O_2 carrying capacity and thus get behind with regards to supply vs. demand! In the pregnancy patient we are oxygenating two patients. By treating the mom's oxygenation status aggressively, we in-turn treat the baby. Therefore, any short-term use of high FiO_2 is good for the patient and won't cause long-term negative affects.

So how do we approach FiO_2 while treating our patients? With the new research out and the trials published by the ARDSNet group, all data is pointing to reduced tidal volumes, higher PEEP and lower FiO_2 concentrations for our ventilator dependent patients. With that being said, I would recommend using enough FiO_2 to maintain a SpO_2 of at least 93%. If that means you turn the FiO_2 down to 30% respectively, then do so. If that means you need to maintain a FiO_2 of 80% for a hypoxic patient to maintain a SpO_2 of 93%, then that's what you do. Obviously, as I have stated above, short-term use of high FiO_2 will not hurt your patient, but I believe that we should practice in the safest means possible and if the patient can maintain sufficient SpO$_2$ ranges above 93% using lower FiO$_2$, then we should be managing our patients in that manner. I lay out a plan on how to optimize lower FiO$_2$ by using PEEP in higher amounts in the PEEP section coming up, which is called the PEEP/FiO$_2$ slide. A chart will be attached in the PEEP section and explained in more detail. Remember, the practice of using lower V$_t$, lower FiO$_2$ and higher amounts of PEEP have been shown to reduce VLI and associated ARDS in our ventilator dependent patients. As such, we shouldn't be causing more harm, but historically we have by being too aggressive with our ventilator volumes and FiO$_2$ strategies.

Trigger (Sensitivity)

When discussing the concept of trigger, or sensitivity, the clinician needs to understand how this applies to the different modes of ventilation. If using a trigger while providing the patient an underlying mode of assist control (AC), you would need to understand how that trigger allows the patient to either take a breath or trigger the ventilator to deliver a breath.

So how does a trigger work and benefit the patient while delivering a pressure or volume breath?

Most ventilators have two triggering options. The primary trigger is the "flow trigger" and it is based on the bias flow. The bias flow is something that is used during the exhalation process to assist with patient triggering. This actually never changes and is then used to set the trigger.

The LTV 1000, 1200, Drager, and ReVel all function a little differently. The lower the number set on the trigger, the lower the volume (ml/sec in a flow trigger) and the lower the pressure (-cmH2O in a pressure trigger), needed for the patient to trigger the ventilator. If the trigger is set higher, the patient will have a more difficult time triggering the ventilator. While flying, the aircraft causes vibrations that can cause problems if using a lower trigger. If you were using assist control (AC) and the vibration caused the trigger to be set off, the patient would be given full tidal volume, multiple breaths, resulting in breath stacking, hyperventilation and cause the patient to become uncomfortable and hypocapnic.

So how does a bias flow of 10L/min work when setting the trigger? If you were to set the trigger at "3", you would in turn be actually setting the trigger at 3L/min. That means that the patient would have to change the flow 3L/min to trigger the ventilator. Now…that may seem like a lot of volume, but actually you have to reduce this down to a more measureable number. Everything we do is in seconds. We would need to reduce the 3L/min down to mL/min and then mL/sec. This is done by a simple calculation.

Example 1:

Bias flow = 3L = 3,000mL/min
1 min = 60 sec
3,000mL/60 sec = 50mL/sec

Example 2:

$$\text{Bias flow} = 5L/min \text{ or } 5{,}000mL/min$$
$$1\ min = 60\ sec$$
$$5000mL/60\ sec = 83ml/sec$$

As I stated above, the bias-flow is a little different for each ventilator. Example, the bias flow set on the LTV 1000, 1200 is 10L/min. In contrast, the bias flow set on the ReVel is defaulted at 5L/min. This means you can only increase your sensitivity to 4 on the Revel, based on the default bias flow of 5L/min. The Hamilton T1 has a bias flow set at 3L/min. You can increase the bias flow on the Revel by changing the setting in the "Vent Control" menu, and increase it up to 10 L/min as well. This would allow you a higher trigger > 4.

Figure 2-2: Example of flow and pressure trigger

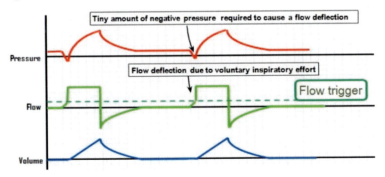

So as you can see from Figure 2-2 above, the patient is drawing 50 mL/sec of flow to tell the ventilator they want to take a breath with the trigger set at (3) respectively. In the transport environment it is important to understand other causes of triggering. Just the vibration of the ambulance or aircraft can cause the ventilator to trigger. It is because of this that we often recommend placing the trigger on a minimum of 3 (3L/min bias flow) and often as high as 5 (5L/min bias flow) depending on the aircraft or road vibration if transporting in an ambulance. What if that is not enough? What if you can't stop the ventilator from auto-triggering in the transport environment? This will depend on the ventilator you use. If it is the LTV1200 you are stuck with using the flow trigger unless you know how to access the pressure trigger in the back menu options. This is done by turning on the "O_2 Conserve" feature. If it is the ReVel you can switch the trigger source from the bias flow trigger to a pressure trigger at the turn of the dial. If you are reading this and scratching your head and wondering what I am talking about, go to your ReVel and turn it on. Once on, place it in the standard volume-SIMV or AC. Then turn your sensitivity dial backward down to (1). Then turn it back one more turn and you will see (P) come up. You have just switched to a pressure trigger. The Revel defaults when you place it in a pressure trigger at (-3 cmH_2O). The bias flow does not turn all the way off. However, it is turned down to 3L/min for purposes of CO_2 removal purposes only. Why -3 cmH_2O? Because anything lower will potentially be too sensitive and auto-triggering may occur as well. This will allow you more control in the transport environment. Why is this better at times? Because any bias-flow trigger is very sensitive to movement. Any change or movement with the circuit that alters or changes the flow will cause auto-triggering. Even you grabbing the vent circuit can cause this change. If the sensitivity is too low it will surely alter the flow and make the ventilator think the patient just triggered a breath. Lastly, "leak" will cause auto-triggering as well. This is actually a big deal and any leak around the ETT cuff can be a significant reason for a triggering event. Remember, once you have a patient sedated or even paralyzed, the trachea and muscles in the neck will change in diameter due to relaxation. It is a slight change, but enough that can cause leak around the ETT cuff. So always evaluate your cuff pressure once the patient is sedated well. This will mitigate any excessive leak phenomenon.

It is also important to allow your patients the ability to take small-triggered breaths. This obviously will depend on their presentation and how much rest they need. However, most studies and research have shown that small amounts of muscle firing are okay and benefit the patient.

Positive End-Expiratory Pressure (PEEP)

Positive end-expiratory pressure (PEEP) is a tool we can use in our ventilator dependent patients to maintain alveolar recruitment and optimize the ability to provide effective oxygenation. It is also one of those things that I find often misunderstood. We have all heard the claims that PEEP significantly reduces venous return and cardiac output, that it has the potential to increase ICP, and that it can cause barotrauma in some patients. Well all of those things are true to a point.

With any treatment or theory in medicine, those most effective are ones that are administered with good critical thinking and in moderation. In addition, understanding the pathophysiology of PEEP and how it can significantly improve your hypoxic patient's oxygenation status in association with the specific disease process is essential in the management of our ventilator dependent patients.

So how much PEEP is good? How much is bad? Well, first it is important to understand that our physiologic PEEP is between 3-5 cmH_2O. If you remember from the section above that talked about absorptive atelectasis, we discussed how when we breathe in atmospheric air it contains 21% oxygen and 78% nitrogen. The nitrogen is very dense and does not diffuse well out of the alveoli. As such, it acts as a pillow and is our internal, physiologic PEEP. Ok...back to our talk on how much PEEP is appropriate. A good starting point for most patients with regards to PEEP is 5 cmH_2O. This gives you good maintenance of alveolar recruitment and is a normal physiologic number.

So what does PEEP really do? Well, often times I hear people say that PEEP recruits alveoli. That just isn't the case. Our alveolar recruitment comes from our inspiratory maneuvers. What does that mean? Well, it is how we administer our tidal volume (V_t). The actual breath that is delivered is how our alveolar units are recruited. Our PEEP maintains that alveoli in an open state at the end of the expiration process. It essentially does not let the alveolar sac deflate. The more PEEP we give, the more the alveoli remain inflated. This is significant when dealing with patients that either have a massive pulmonary shunt or have alveoli that are already brittle and can't handle collapse. This is called atelectasis.

So now that we have an understanding of how PEEP works and the importance of maintaining alveolar recruitment, let's discuss the different strategies used with PEEP based on different presentations. As I stated above, PEEP is the tool used in association with FiO_2 to maintain adequate oxygenation. As we have discussed in the previous section on FiO_2, using high concentrations of oxygen can lead to oxygen toxicity and the release of free radials that attack our lung tissues. Because of this, we need to maintain the absolute lowest FiO_2 possible. We can safely do this by using PEEP as an augmentation tool. By using lower FiO_2 and higher PEEP, we decrease the possibility of oxygen toxicity and oxygenate our patients very effectively. Now I am not saying that we need 10-15 cmH_2O for every patient. However, what I am saying is that we may need to use a PEEP of 5-8 cmH_2O on most patients. This is just fine and is more beneficial to our patients in the long run. Remember, oxygen toxicity is very harmful, leads to massive inflammatory cascades and starts the processes that lead to ARDS. Below is a great tool that you can use to optimize oxygenation by providing a low FiO_2 and the use of PEEP to provide excellent oxygenation. In proceeding charts, you will see that you can use very low FiO_2 and moderate PEEP to maintain oxygenation and alveolar recruitment.

PEEP/FiO₂ slide:

Oxygenation goal: PaO$_2$ 55-80 mmHg or SpO$_2$ 88-94%

Lower PEEP/FiO₂ table

FiO$_2$	0.3	0.4	0.4	0.5	0.5	0.6	0.7	0.7	0.7
PEEP	5	5	8	8	10	10	10	12	14

FiO$_2$	0.8	0.9	0.9	0.9	1.0
PEEP	14	14	16	18	18-24

As you can see from the above chart, you will use higher PEEP in combination with lower FiO$_2$. Most often, you will be able to oxygenate your patients appropriately using a FiO$_2$ in the 0.5 range and PEEP of 8 cmH$_2$O respectively.

In later sections we will discuss the two different strategies we can use to treat our ventilator dependent patients. Those two strategies are the injury approach and the obstructive approach. I bring this up now because it is important to understand that using PEEP in each of these strategies will be completely different. In the injury approach (any patient that does not have COPD or asthma), your patients may need PEEP that starts at 5 cmH$_2$O and you could increase based on the patient's oxygenation status into the 20 cmH$_2$O range. Now those high PEEP numbers are often only seen in patients with massive shunt, like an ARDS patient. The obstructive approach is reserved for only patients suffering from either COPD or asthma. Obstruction of the airways and alveoli is what is occurring. Those patients are not usually suffering from hypoxia. If they are hypoxic, it is most often due to the poor vital capacity per breath they are able to take because of the obstructive properties of the disease. Remember, this is a disease that causes ventilatory failure, essentially an inability to regulate CO_2. They are in a profound ventilation failure. That means that they are unable to exhale properly causing a build up of gases in the chest and alveolar sacs. This is called air trapping and this phenomenon then progresses into auto-PEEP. Because of the auto-PEEP phenomenon, if you were to add more PEEP to this patient, it would significantly add to the problem and hinder them even more. It would lead to reduced chest wall compliance, a reduction of venous return and higher plateau pressures (Pplat).

So how do we know how much auto-PEEP a patient currently has? Most ventilators have a function called an expiratory hold button. This will allow the clinician the ability to identify the patient's current auto-PEEP. To perform this maneuver, the clinician needs to make sure the PEEP is completely turned off. Then by pushing and holding the expiratory hold button, you will be able to identify the patient's current auto-PEEP. For example, you have a patient that has an exacerbation of COPD and you identify an auto-PEEP of 12 cmH_2O. By adding the standard starting 5 cmH_2O of additional PEEP to this patient, you are going to decrease their ability to exhale even more and your patient will decompensate quicker. So how much do we give in the obstructive patient. Well, it is recommended to stay between 0-3 cmH_2O and to never exceed 3 cmH_2O. We will revisit the obstructive and injury approach in greater detail later in the book. I just wanted to illustrate the importance of understanding how the patient's disease process can significantly change your approach when administering PEEP.

PEEP is a tool that we need to understand when using our ventilator. It is a tool that will greatly improve shunt, V/Q mismatch and reduce the incidence of atelectasis trauma. Understanding the significant benefits as it relates to the PEEP/FiO_2 slide as well as the different patient presentations that can make PEEP administration beneficial or harmful is essential. PEEP is your friend; so don't forget to utilize it when it is needed.

Pressure Support (PS)

When using synchronized intermittent mandatory ventilation (SIMV), pressure support is used to help your patient take a triggered spontaneous breath. This is essentially an augmentation pressure that is applied to the end of the ventilator circuit to reduce dead space and thus reduce the workload on the patient during those spontaneous breaths.

Pressure support (PS) is a pressure-targeted mode of ventilation support. Each inspiratory effort by the patient while using SIMV is augmented by an elevation in airway pressure at the onset of an inspiratory effort. This elevation in airway pressure is termed the pressure support level and is preset to a level that will decrease the work of breathing. The pressure support is maintained through inspiration, and is discontinued when the inspiratory flow falls and expiration begins.

So how much PS do we use? Your starting point should always be 10 cmH$_2$O, but any changes up or down need only be by 1 cmH$_2$O at a time. 1 cmH$_2$O will equal 75-150 mL of augmented ability in V$_t$. You can see that the PS is very sensitive and we do not want our patients taking too much. This allows for a greater gradient and gives the patient a more optimal pressure while taking spontaneous breaths while on SIMV. There have been several studies that evaluated the optimal PS levels needed. *Brochard and colleagues* evaluated different levels of PS and assessed diaphragmatic fatigue. They identified that using 10-20 cmH$_2$O of PS prevented impending fatigue 7 out of 8 times (Brochard et al., 1989). In addition, the study concluded that using PS could be used to decrease the work of breathing caused by an endotracheal tube and the ventilator circuit respectively.

Remember, we want our patients taking some spontaneous breaths, but we do not want them to overwork. Maintaining a maximum of 75% of the desired V$_t$ based on their IBW is the key. If they were exceeding this during spontaneous breaths, then you would increase their pain and sedation treatment and decrease their PS by 1 cmH$_2$O.

When providing mechanical ventilation and using SIMV as your mode of ventilation, PS is always used to augment the patient's spontaneously triggered breath. Using a PS level of 10 cmH$_2$O as a starting number is recommended. This will reduce the work of breathing associated with the increased dead space seen by the endotracheal tube and ventilator circuit. The PS level should be titrated to increase the patient's spontaneous V_t and to decrease the patient's respiratory rate. This level of pressure support should allow the patient's spontaneous V_t to reach no more than 75% of your set ventilated controlled Vt that is based on ideal body weight. So what does that mean? Imagine you identified an ideal body weight of 70 kg and you set your V_t at 400 mL. By using PS to augment the patient's spontaneous V_t, you would not allow that patient to take a spontaneous V_t of 75% of that set controlled Vt, so that would be no more than 300 mL of V_t during the patients spontaneous breath. Why? We do not want to allow the patient to work too hard. This is a simple combination of pain management using Fentanyl and sedation using small aliquots of Versed, Valium or ketamine.

Remember, they are sick and have sick lungs. We use the SIMV mode of ventilation with the addition of PS to allow the patient some comfort and ability to fire those respiratory muscles. For that reason, all the studies are demonstrating that SIMV is more beneficial than assist control when managing our ventilator dependent patients. I will discuss this in more depth during our modes of ventilation section.

PS is a great tool to use when providing ventilation using SIMV. Lastly, it is important to understand that your PS is actually your PS + PEEP. Why? Because your PEEP is maintained constantly throughout both the inhalation and exhalation phases. This means that if you have a PEEP 5 cmH_2O and a PS 10 cmH_2O, your PS in reality is 15 cmH_2O. That being said, raising your PS in smaller increments as I have stated above is the best solution. There is also no need to raise your PS every time your PEEP is increased. If PEEP is moved to 10 cmH$_2$O, and PS is currently set at 10 cmH$_2$O, essentially now you have a PEEP 10 and a PS 20 respectively (**Refer to the BiPAP section on Additive vs. Absolute for starting PS example and expanded explanation**). The more PS we apply, the easier is will be for the patient to take a spontaneously triggered breath in SIMV. It is an excellent tool and will benefit your patients greatly!

Peak Inspiratory Pressure (PIP)

The peak inspiratory pressure (PIP) is measured at the peak of inspiration and is a representation of many factors. It is a measurement of the volume of each breath, compliance of the lungs, airway resistance and the force needed to deliver the breath. The vent uses a formula to determine this pressure and will give the clinician this pressure second-by-second. Most ventilators have this pressure recorded in two different locations; often a bar graph at the top of the ventilator and then as a numerical value in the settings screen.

High pressure will have a direct affect on VLI, however has no significant relationship to alveolar function or physiology. For this reason we want our PIP to stay <35 cmH$_2$O. The PIP is one of two important pressures we monitor on every patient. It is also the highest pressure at all times on the ventilator. The second pressure we monitor, and actually the most important pressure out of the two, is the plateau pressure (P$_{plat}$). We will dive into that in the next section, however it is important to point out a few rules when looking at the PIP and P$_{plat}$.

Figure 2-3: Example of an inspiratory waveform

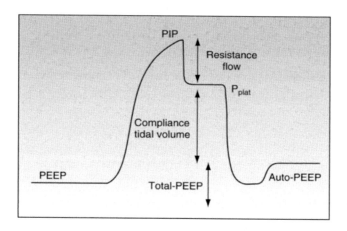

Rule #1: Increased PIP and unchanged P$_{plat}$ represents pressure limited by airway resistance and not an indication of alveolar health or pressure.

Rationale:

If we have our flow rate set to deliver the breath quicker (over 0.5 sec vs. 1 sec), it will affect your PIP in a negative way and drive this pressure higher. Patients with increased airway resistance (i.e. asthma, COPD) will have higher and prolonged PIP. We also need to always consider a kinked ETT, vent circuit, patients needing suctioning, patients needing sedation, and patients over breathing the ventilator.

Rule #2: Increased PIP and increased P$_{plat}$ represents pressure elevated in the alveolar spaces and lower lung

fields. The PIP being elevated is due mostly by the transient pressure being forced upward from the lower airways.

Rationale:

Plateau pressures are a direct indication of alveolar function. Consistently high plateau pressures will lead to alveolar destruction and VLI contributing to ARDS and inflammatory cascades that can increase the risk of death. Anytime you see your PIP increase, you need to then immediately identify if your P_{plat} has increased and whether this is the primary cause. I will go into all things P_{plat} in the next section.

Plateau Pressure (P_{plat})

As mentioned above, plateau pressures are a direct indication of alveolar function. Consistently high plateau pressures will lead to alveolar destruction and VLI contributing to ARDS and inflammatory cascades that can increase the risk of death. As such, our treatment goal plateau pressure is <30 cmH$_2$O to prevent barotrauma; lung injury secondary to over distension of alveoli.

In patients without lung disease, peak inspiratory pressure (PIP) is only slightly higher than the plateau pressure. In cases of increased tidal volume or decreased pulmonary compliance, the PIP and P_{plat} rise together proportionately. If the peak pressure rises with no change in plateau pressure, increased airway resistance should be suspected or high inspiratory gas flow.

Your plateau pressure waveform will change based on the inspiratory pause time. The ideal inspiratory hold is 0.5 sec, in which you hold down the inspiratory hold button for 0.5 sec.

Figure 2-4: Example of PIP and P$_{plat}$ waveform

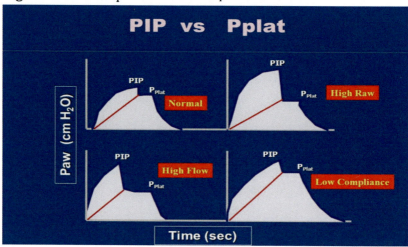

(Nickson, n.d.)

Causes of high P$_{plat}$ >30 cmH$_2$O:

- Increased tidal volume
- Decreased pulmonary compliance
- Pulmonary edema
- Pleural effusion
- Peritoneal gas insufflation
- Tension pneumothorax
- Trendelenburg
- Ascites
- Abdominal packing

How do we decrease a high P_{plat}? Why is it important? Remember, an over-stretched alveolus is mad! It will send out distress signals. These distress signals stimulate cytokines. These are little red flags that attract neutrophils and inflammatory cells. These cells attack first and ask questions later and cause all sorts of damage. They damage type II pneumocytes that cause reduced surfactant, and in the end lead to atelectasis trauma and increased vascular permeability, which is the precursor to ARDS. The reduction of P_{plat} into normal ranges should always be your first and primary objective. The best approach is to remember three simple steps and attempt to reduce the P_{plat} using these rules.

Rule #1: Always attempt to identify the pathophysiology behind a high (> 30 cmH$_2$O) P_{plat}. Is this increased pressure a result of a tension pneumothorax? Is this simply a result of ARDS and high alveolar-capillary pressures? If it is something you can correct now, then do it. The tension pneumothorax presentation would be immediately treated with chest decompression on the affected side.

Rule #2: Volume will always play into how much alveolar pressure is being seen and measured. Because of this, V_t is a big player in our P_{plat} and will be the single most significant determining factor in increasing or decreasing this pressure. We always first identify if there is a pathophysiology issue (as stated in step 1 above), but quickly move to identify if the Vt is causing this increased pressure. Remember our lung protective strategy. We start our V_t range at 6-8 mL/kg, with the most ideal starting number at 6 mL/kg. If you had a patient with a starting range of 6 mL/kg and they were 100kg of ideal body weight, your V_t would be 600 mL. You would then start decreasing your V_t from 6mL/kg down to 5mL/kg and the corresponding V_t of 500 mL for that patient's ideal body weight. You then re-evaluate your P_{plat} by doing the 0.5 sec inspiratory hold and identify if the reduction in Vt had any corresponding effect on the P_{plat}. In this scenario, you would continue to do this until you reached 4 mL/kg of Vt and lowered the patient's V_t to the corresponding V_t of 400 mL. Again, re-evaluating the P_{plat} as stated above. Now, at this point if you still don't have your P_{plat} at a level <30 cmH_2O, then your patient's presentation may be such that other measures may be needed. We will discuss this in the next rule.

Rule #3: If the above measures have not taken care of reducing the P_{plat}, you need to remember that there can be many other causes:

       a. Increased tidal volume
       b. Decreased pulmonary compliance
       c. Pulmonary edema
       d. Pleural effusion
       e. Tension pneumothorax
       f. Trendelenburg
       g. Ascites
       h. Abdominal packing

As such, steps need to be taken to identify if you can correct anything from the above list. Most often, these *issues have been looked at and attempts have been made to correct them. With that being said, your next step in reducing the P_{plat} is to move the patient from a volume delivered breath to a pressure delivered breath. Pressure control ventilation is a great mode of delivery that is based on lung compliance. We will dissect this later in the book and tie this together.*

Mean Airway Pressure (MAP)

Mean airway pressure (MAP) is the average pressure exerted on the airways and lungs from the beginning of inspiration to the beginning of the next inspiration. Unfortunately, this measurement on your ventilator is something that many clinicians miss and often do not understand its significance. It truly is the most powerful influence on oxygenation. Essentially, our mean airway pressure is all about your ability to oxygenate. This concept is very simple. Think of alveolar recruitment and the overall amount of volume that can fill the airways without causing over-distention, increased P_{plat} and barotrauma. So with that being said, increased PIP, total PEEP, inspiratory time, (f), and inspiratory flow patterns will all affect your mean airway pressure. Your goal is to maintain a MAP of <12 cmH_2O, as levels above that range can contribute to barotrauma. With that being said, there are patients that need >12 cmH_2O to maintain alveolar recruitment and oxygenation due to their underlying disease process. Additionally, modes of ventilation such as Airway Pressure Release Ventilation (APRV), High Frequency Ventilation (HOF), CPAP and BiPAP all focus on raising MAP to optimize alveolar recruitment and corresponding oxygenation potential. These patients will need augmentation of their hemodynamic status with vasopressors to maintain an adequate hemodynamic status.

MAP calculation formula:

PIP = Peak inspiratory pressure
IT = Inspiratory time
PEEP = Positive end expiratory pressure
ET = Expiratory time

MAP = (PIP * % IT) + (PEEP * % ET)

The great thing about this formula is that we can rely on our ventilator to give us that number. Remember, your goal is to always provide an adequate MAP but not to exceed 12 cmH$_2$O. Obviously your PEEP and inspiratory time will be the greatest tool in optimizing your oxygenation potential.

Delta Pressure (Delta P)

The delta pressure (Delta P) is a parameter comprised of the difference between PIP and PEEP (PIP − PEEP). The significance of this number is two-fold. First, this is the technique used to identify your starting inspiratory pressure when using pressure control ventilation (PCV). Obviously we use this as a guide and stop at a level that won't cause alveolar damage and barotrauma, but it is a tool that will get you to a good starting pressure for pressure initiated-volume targeted Vt. The standard stopping point would be 35 cmH$_2$O.

An example of this would be a patient with chronic asthma and exacerbation with a consistently high PIP of 50 cmH$_2$O. If we had this patient on a PEEP of 5 cmH$_2$O and use the formula I stated above (PIP – PEEP), we would have a delta P of 45 cmH$_2$O. Even though this may seem high, it is relevant to the patient's chronic disease process. If that does not make a lot of sense now, the second reason we use this should add some clarity to the above scenario.

Driving Pressure

The second, and most important aspect is what is called "driving pressure". Your driving pressure must be equal to the opening pressure to open and ventilate the alveoli. The addition of PEEP decreases opening pressure by increasing the diameter of the alveoli and thus increasing the surface tension. Less driving pressure is needed to ventilate the lungs.

Driving pressure has become a common concept in the past year, with the new goal for patients with ALI or ARDS having a driving pressure <15 cmH$_2$O. A resent study by ***Amato et al., Driving Pressure and Survival in the Acute Respiratory Distress Syndrome***, identified morbidity and mortality increase in patients with driving pressures >15 cmH$_2$O. How do we decrease driving pressure? Driving pressure is the difference between V$_t$ and static compliance. So your driving pressure is your (Pplat − PEEP). This takes our Pplat goal of <30 cmH$_2$O and really throws it out the window. Example: Your patient has a current Pplat 25 cmH$_2$O and PEEP 5 cmH$_2$O. This would be a driving pressure of 20 cmH$_2$O. This is significant in the ALI or ARDS patient. We need to either lower our Pplat or increase our PEEP. To lower our Pplat, we lower our Vt. We can lower our Vt down to 4 mL/kg and evaluate our Pplat with each 1 mL/kg drop in Vt. We can also bring down our driving pressure by increasing our PEEP. In the end, this theory is only applicable for those ALI and ARDS patient. In a normal healthy lung, there is no set driving pressure. We all have different driving pressures and shouldn't worry about this for other non-lung injured patients.

Dead Space

Dead space is the amount of volume lost that does not reach the alveolar level during each mechanically delivered breath. It is measured in milliliters (mL) and is lost in multiple areas. We see this most significantly in the ventilator circuit, ETT (mechanical dead space), and anatomical locations (bronchioles, lung units). Why is this significant? When we look at overall minute ventilation, we are attempting to match our physiological levels. Those levels are between 4-8 L/min. However, we need to understand that when delivering a breath via the ventilator, all that volume does not reach the alveolar-capillary membrane for gas exchange. This can be a really big issue and often causes hypoventilation and poor eucapnia. The key concept here is identifying actual alveolar minute ventilation and not just overall minute ventilation delivered by the ventilator. There is a big difference between the two. How much do we potentially lose? There are two ways to calculate this. The textbook answer is to calculate this by 1mL/1 pound of ideal body weight. For an adult patient that most often is approximately 150mL per breath. However, with anyone under 70kg or 150 pounds it is best to use the 1mL/1 pound of ideal body weight formula.

Let's examine this further. Our new strategy involving lung protection actually may cause an increase in dead space ventilation. This may also add to intrathoracic pressure and impede venous return. Why? Smaller breaths have a higher percentage of dead space, which adds to intrathoracic pressure but does not participate in gas exchange. Thus, for a given ventilation need (alveolar ventilation, or the volume that actually exchanges CO_2 and O_2), it is more efficient to use larger and much slower breaths when dealing with dead space. However! This is not saying that we stop using lung protective strategies. We just need to understand the impact it makes on our patients. This probably does not make a huge difference when comparing 8/min to 12/min, but this is gigantic when you look at intrathoracic pressures with rates of 20-30/min (which are incredibly common). When we look at a patient that is suffering from ARDS and compare them with a patient suffering from multi-system trauma with hemodynamic collapse, this may be a major factor in our patient's ability to compensate and stay in an optimal perfusion state.

Let's look at this from the trauma aspect. It may give you more clarity. One of the newest strategies for ventilation in the trauma patient with hemodynamic instability is to deliver high Vt and low rates based on the study, *A structural model of perfusion and oxygenation in low-flow states,* conducted by (Davis & Davis 2011). Based on that literature, 10-12mL/kg is employed, with respiratory rates of 6-8/min, in the hopes of decreasing dead space and overall intrathoracic pressure.

One thing to realize about this "hypotensive approach" is that there is a point where the larger tidal volumes actually add more to intrathoracic pressure than they contribute to gas exchange. However, this does not occur until the "upper inflection point" is reached.

What's the "upper inflection point"? That is the maximum amount of volume our lungs can handle before we see barotrauma. In a normal set of lungs, that is not until 1.5-2 liters (way more than we would be giving). However, for ARDS (which is where most ventilator recommendations are derived), the upper inflection point can be much less than a liter. That is how we reconcile our recommendations for larger/slower breaths against the "lung-protective" strategies (which were derived for ARDS) that use smaller/faster breaths. They are actually very compatible when you consider the upper inflection point being much lower in ARDS. In addition, the primary challenge in ARDS is oxygenation due to the diseased lungs and oxygen being perfusion-dependent. In other words, it may be worth the hemodynamic compromise from elevated intrathoracic pressure to avoid hypoxia in

ARDS. In a bleeding trauma patient, this may not be true (Davis & Davis, 2011).

Based on all these different aspects, how do we treat our patients? How do we maintain the proper alveolar minute ventilation that is purposeful and indeed accounts for gas exchange? The best way is to employ the easy to remember formula we discussed in the above section on minute ventilation. By employing the formula, 100mL/kg/min, you will account for that dead space loss and maintain adequate alveolar minute ventilation.

Lastly, how do we account for mechanical dead space? Very easy! Each ventilator circuit will have an exact number associated with potential loss. But for easy math we can use the below formula to identify the dead space loss in an adult and pediatric vent circuit. What is the cut off with an adult circuit vs. a pediatric circuit with regards to age?

- Adult Ventilator Circuit: > 20 kg
- Pediatric Ventilator Circuit: < 20 kg

Ventilator circuit dead space formula:

- Adult circuit: 2mL x PIP
    - **Example: PIP = 30 cmH$_2$O**
    - 2mL x 30 = **60 mL (dead space loss)**
- Pediatric circuit: 1 mL x PIP
    - **Example: PIP = 18 cmH$_2$O**
    - 1mL x 18 = **18 mL (dead space loss)**

Ideal Body Weight (IBW)

Ideal body weight is something that is very important to calculate on any patient we place on the ventilator. We always need to remember that the lung protective strategies we employ are only as good as our understanding of body weight or "ideal body weight"! The concept here is simple. If you have a male patient that is 5'11" in height and has an actual body weight of 350-pounds, we know his lung capacity is not of a 350-pound person, it is actually based on his height. A 350-pound person would calculate to 160 kg. This would give a V_t of 960mL. Obviously this is crazy when using the lung protective strategies we now use. In actuality, we would identify his height and then calculate his IBW based on that. This gives us a closer representation of actual lung capacity and allows for a better representation of physiologic V_t.

Now, I know there are different ways to calculate IBW, but I am all about doing things as simply and quickly as possible. Many use calculations of (2.3) per inch in their formulas. That seems counter-productive to me, as we often round our patient weight up anyway and this is our objective assessment on height regardless. So essentially it is a crapshoot! We are not taking out a tape measure and measuring someone. So who really cares about (2.3); lets use (2) instead!

Based on that same patient, see below for the following calculation. You will see that the formula starts with a standard height of 5'0" and a weight of 50 kg. That means that a 5'0" person should have an IBW of 50 kg. From there all we do is now estimate their height. If your patient is 5'11", then you take the inches above your standard starting 5'0" and multiply that by (2). You then take that number which would be 11 x 2 = 22 and then add that to your starting weight of 50 kg. 50kg + 22kg = 77kg IBW. Now from there I would again round my answer down or up to the nearest 10 based on simple rounding math. In this case I would round up and use an IBW of 80kg.

Calculation: 5'0" = 50 kg
Then multiply 2 times every inch above 5'0" of estimated height of the pt.
So??? A 5'__10__" male would look like this.
10 inches x 2 = 20 + 50 kg = 70 kg
Round up or down to nearest 10's = 70kg IBW
70 kg x 6-8 cc/kg = 420 – 560 V_t

See the example chart below that compares (2.3) & (2) as our multiplier. Make the math easy for yourself!

Height	Inch's > 60"	Multiple by (2)	IBW Result (Round)	Multiplied by (2.3)	IBW Result (Round)
5'3"	3	6	56/60	6.9	56.9/60
5'6"	6	12	62/60	13.8	63.8/60
5'10"	10	20	70	23	73/70
6'2"	14	28	78/80	32.2	82.2/80
6'6"	18	36	86/90	41.4	91.4/90

Chapter 3 – Modes of Ventilation

Volume Initiated Ventilation

Volume-targeted (initiated) ventilation is our standard starting manner of delivery. This involves the simple concept of filling the lung with a set amount of volume. That volume is determined by identifying the patient's IBW and using the calculation formula of 4-8mL/kg based on our lung protective strategies. Although this manner of delivery is simple and targeted, it can lead to barotrauma and increased plateau pressures (Pplat) if administered in high amounts. For purposes of definition only, we will not go into that part during this section because we discussed that in-depth during the section on plateau pressures.

Pressure Initiated Ventilation

In contrast to volume-targeted ventilation, pressure ventilation is said to be volume targeted-pressure regulated. This manner of delivery is different than volume delivery in that the volume delivered is dependent on lung compliance. With that being said, you are now essentially blowing up a "balloon" to a set pressure. Based on that pressure and the overall lung compliance you will get a volume. The tidal volume is determined by the preset pressure limit, which is set based off your delta pressure (PIP – PEEP), not to exceed 35 cmH$_2$O, and is a peak pressure rather than a plateau pressure limit (easier to measure). With that being said, make it simple! It is much easier to start at a Pinsp of 20 cmH$_2$O for adults and 10-15 cmH$_2$O for neonates and pediatrics. As the airway pressure rises with increasing alveolar volume, the rate of flow drops off until a point is reached when the delivered pressure equals the airway pressure flow.

Pressure ventilation is the best manner of delivery for many reasons. As I illustrated above, this is a compliance-based mode and will be very gentle on sick "baby" lungs. Most of our patients that are ventilator dependent have these classic "baby" lungs. Volume targeted-pressure delivered breaths will protect those lungs and allow for lower P_{plat} pressures and reduce barotrauma potential. For these reasons, this manner of delivery has been the go-to mode of delivery for our neonates and pediatric population for years.

Rise Time

When we use pressure ventilation as the way we deliver a breath we have a feature that many providers either forget to utilize or maybe do not even understand. So what is rise time? Rise time is a tool we use in pressure delivery to either shorten or lengthen the time it takes to deliver the breath. So, what is the difference in I-time vs. your Rise time? Imagine taking a trip with your family to Disney world. Rise time is the amount of time it takes to drive to Disney world. In contrast, I-time is the amount of time you stay at Disney world. Based on that analogy, rise time can be a very powerful tool for patients that are challenging to manage. How do you access rise time? Pushing and holding down the "select" button on the top of the ventilator where the screen is located will allow you to access the back menu. Scroll through once this menu comes up and find "Ventilator Control" ("Vent Op" in LTV). You will see "Rise Time", with nine different profiles. The LTV 1000, 1200 and ReVel ventilators for example default to a rise time of (4). The Hamilton T1 uses RAMP via a percentage, to adjust Rise time. How does Rise Time work? As I stated above, there are nine different profiles. Each profile will add 33% to the length of the delivery. See below for the examples based on time in (seconds) for each profile.

Rise Time Profiles:

Profile 1 = 0.100 sec
Profile 2 = 0.133 sec
Profile 3 = 0.178 sec
Profile 4 = 0.237 sec
Profile 5 = 0.316 sec
Profile 6 = 0.422 sec
Profile 7 = 0.562 sec
Profile 8 = 0.750 sec
Profile 9 = 1.000 sec

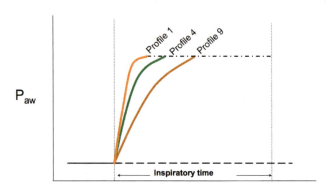

Slower Rise time (Profile 5-9) is desired for: small ETT, bronchospasm, pressure overshoot. Faster Rise time is

desired for patient needing fast inspiratory time. Think of patients that are hypoxic and air starved.

As you can see, the **Profile 1** will deliver the breath over 0.1 sec or a tenth of a second. This is very fast. You can use this for a patient that is air hungry, with associated hypoxia. In addition some patients need a higher V_t due to poor compliance, with associated high peak inspiratory pressures (PIP). In this type of patient, it may be better to deliver the breath faster. A lower Rise time profile will give you a larger V_t. This is important to understand, as you can raise and lower your patient's V_t according to your Rise time profile change. In contrast, imagine a patient in ARDS that needs longer recruitment times. The **Profile 9** would be great for those patients that need consistent recruitment due to severe shunt (ARDS, Pneumonia), with the breath given over 1 second. However, remember your increased Rise time profile will then decrease the total V_t. If this does not make sense, go place your ventilator on a test lung, place it in PCV and then identify your V_{te}. Change your Rise time profile to (1), then look at your V_{te}. You will see that your V_{te} has increased. Then change it to a Rise time **Profile 9**. You will then see a huge change in the opposite direction and should see a lower V_{te}.

Flow Termination

Flow termination is something that many do not have a clear understanding of. If you are just trying to figure out more basic aspects of mechanical ventilation, the last thing you have been studying is flow termination.

However, flow termination is a very important part of cycling from inspiration to expiration on a ventilator driven or spontaneous breath, with Pressure Control (PC) flow termination controlling PCV breaths and flow termination controlling spontaneous (PS) breaths as seen with SIMV or NPPV (BiPAP).

Many ventilators will have the flow termination preset at 25% of peak flow. Based on this, if the peak flow on a spontaneous breath was 100 L/min, inspiration would proceed until the flow from the ventilator decreased or decelerated to 25% of its initial level. In this example, that would be 25 L/min. Basically, the deceleration of flow by the ventilator is a response to patient demand. As the patient's demand decreases, flow decelerates, and based on the flow termination setting, inspiration is then terminated. With that being said, the lower the flow termination %, the more potential V_t is available from breath to breath.

See Figure 3-1 for an example. You will note the different flow termination % settings available on most ventilators. The Carefusion LTV1200 and REVEL go from 40% down to 10%. The Hamilton T1 goes from 80% down to 0%.

Figure 3-1

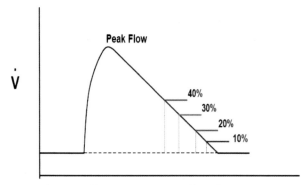

Note: At 40% your flow is terminated and inspiration is then terminated. Also note the area under the curve. That is all V_t. However, look at 10% and notice there is more area under the curve. That means the V_t potential is greater. So, a lower flow termination % gives you a higher V_t potential. The vertical line from that point is then the start of exhalation.

This feature provides a means to adjust the termination of spontaneous inspiration based on the peak flow. This will directly affect the patient's overall spontaneous V_t. Let's imagine we want our patient to have larger spontaneous V_t. A longer spontaneous inspiratory time would then be desirable. Flow termination would be set at 10% and inspiration would continue until the flow decelerated down to 10 L/min (10% of 100 L/min).

Figure 3-2

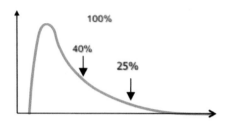

Flow termination set at 25% is going to be accurate for most of your patients.

Figure 3-3

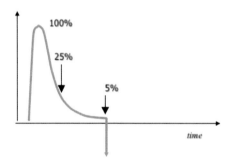

In ARDS, due to the low compliance, the inspiratory flow rapidly decelerates. The usual 25% might lead to an extremely short inspiratory time. We know this will be the opposite of what an ARDS patient needs. Move the flow termination to 10% in these types of patients.

Figure 3-4

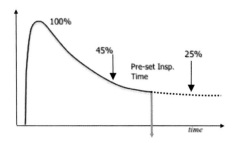

High airway resistance may prevent the inspiratory flow to drop fast enough to reach the termination point in tolerable inspiratory times.

Time Termination

Time termination is another function that is often missed with clinical providers as they learn the initial application of mechanical ventilation. Time termination is applied to spontaneous pressure support (PS) breaths. So this means PS breaths while in SIMV or in the application of NPPV/BiPAP. We need to always adjust the time termination to be at, or a little higher, than what we have the patients I-time set to. It makes no sense to have an I-time of 1.0 sec for example and have your time termination, which often is defaulted on ventilator start-up at 2.0 seconds. So in this example, turning your time termination from the defaulted 2.0 seconds, down to 1.0-1.2 seconds, will match your set I-time of 1.0 second with any spontaneous PS breaths. To make this even more simple, we do not want our mandatory control breaths terminated at 1.0 second based on your set I-time and then having any spontaneous PS breaths terminated at 2.0

seconds based on your default time termination setting. Always make your time termination match or be a little higher than your I-time! Lastly, this needs to be set anytime you are using SIMV with PS or NPPV modes of ventilation.

Assist Control (AC)

Assist control (AC) is a mode that many clinicians working in the hospital setting are familiar with. It has been the standard mode of ventilation for years and has proven to be very effective in delivering set minute ventilations for patients needing respiratory rest that we can adequately treat for pain and sedation. This mode is also great for those asthma or COPD patients that have ventilation failure.

AC has some primary characteristics that we will discuss. First, AC will deliver a set Vt and RR based on what the clinician enters into the ventilator settings. It guarantees this for every breath. This is accomplished in both volume targeted and pressure targeted modes of delivery. AC also allows the patient to trigger a breath based on the trigger we set. As we discussed in the section on trigger in chapter 2, the amount of sensitivity we set based on the bias flow allows the patient the ability to trigger a breath. In the context of AC, the ventilator then senses this need and then delivers a full (mandatory) Vt breath. That means if we have the Vt set at 400mL, every time the patient triggers a breath, it will then deliver a full Vt breath of 400mL.

My view on AC is multi-layered. I believe this mode is great for the ICU setting and allows the patient the ability to be ventilated appropriately. However, in the transport environment, I believe that AC has its issues. Keep in mind that this is my view and only my view. I have had many discussions with respiratory therapists on this subject with most agreeing, however with some disagreeing. With that being said, I have seen these problems throughout my 15 years in HEMS-Critical Care and have to say that I believe my thoughts and strategies regarding AC to be sound.

In the transport environment we have many additional limitations that are not experienced in the hospital setting. ICU's are quiet, dark, and have a level of control that the transport environment does not have. In the ICU you can easily assess your patient, identify their pain and sedation status easier and quicker than in a dark, noisy helicopter or ground ambulance. In addition, the vibration aspect of transport adds a completely different dimension on your ventilation strategies. It is not uncommon to see patients being hyperventilated on AC because of mismanagement of the trigger setting alone. The aircraft or ambulance vibration causes the ventilator to think the patient is attempting to trigger a breath. Due to this, the ventilator will then continually give full assisted breaths based off what it thinks is the patient triggering a breath. This not only causes significant stress on the patient, but will also lead to air-trapping and auto-PEEP issues, poor compliance and poor eucapnia. Couple this with our inability to truly identify our patient's sedation and pain status early and you have a patient that is now in even more pain. Lastly, hospital ventilators are much more sophisticated and equipped with added technologies that the transport ventilator does not have. Most hospital ventilators have features that will not allow another triggered breath while in AC until a set time period as been met. This limits any auto-triggering and helps deliver the set Vt and rate as they were set to do. Again, our transport ventilators do not have this added technology.

Imagine being aware of everything and having the ventilator give full Vt breaths over and over. This would be terrible. It is because of this phenomenon that I do not use AC and go straight to synchronized intermittent mandatory ventilation (SIMV) for my patients while in transport. Obviously there are uses for AC and it has been proven to be a great mode of ventilation, and one that is still widely used. However, I believe that SIMV, if used correctly, will benefit your patients more and really enhance your ability to care for these patients in the transport environment.

In the end, there are many different views out there on which mode of ventilation is the best, with most believing that pressure regulated volume control (PRVC) is the best (we will discuss this later in this chapter). I believe the trend is moving towards more intensivists using SIMV over AC for the fact of wanting their patients driving some respiratory effort and taking small V_t breaths. I think this is limited to the most progressive teaching hospitals and do not see this trend throughout the United States. Obviously over time this will either become the trend or will die out. Regardless, I believe if I have a choice between the two I will always pick SIMV.

Synchronized Intermittent Mandatory Ventilation (SIMV)

Synchronized intermittent mandatory ventilation (SIMV) is my go-to mode of ventilation. I think this is an excellent all around mode of ventilation that allows the clinician to augment the patient's attempt to initiate his or her own breath. This in turn starts the weaning process and is a very comfortable mode for the patient. There are many similar characteristics with SIMV when compared to AC. However, there are a few additional tools that SIMV affords you that are beneficial for patient care and for overall treatment strategies.

SIMV allows you to set guaranteed minute ventilation by setting a V_t and RR. In addition, it allows you to set the trigger using the strategies we discussed in chapter 2. However, instead of the ventilator giving a full V_t breath as we have learned with AC, SIMV will allow the patients to take their own V_t breath. This is based on many factors including pain and sedation status predominantly, but gives the patient the ability to have a small sense of control. With that being said, once the patient triggers the breath based on the set flow trigger (or pressure trigger if used), the patient will be able to take a V_t breath based on their current respiratory status, sedation and pain level. If they do not trigger a spontaneous breath within the respiratory cycle time then the ventilator will give an assisted breath. This is a mandatory breath per your set V_t if in VCV or pressure if in PCV. In addition, SIMV allows us to augment a patient's spontaneous breath by using a tool called pressure support (PS). Do not get this confused with pressure control. I see that often. Those are completely different terms. We have discussed PS in chapter 2 and the strategies involved with employing this tool. However, for recap purposes, it is best to set your PS at least 5-10 cmH_2O above your PEEP. The more PS you add, the easier it will be for your patients to take a spontaneous breath based on the set flow trigger. Essentially PS is used to reduce the (dead space) workload while the patient is taking a triggered spontaneous breath.

Remember, a good starting PS is 10 cmH_2O (remember, know your ventilator – additive or absolute). Based on that number, you will then evaluate the patient's V_{te} and identify if the PS is allowing the patient too much added effort in their spontaneous V_t or too little. You can use the analogy of a milk shake and sucking out of a straw to represent PS. If your pressure support is inadequate think of this as you sucking a very thick milk shake out of a straw. As you add PS, think about thinning the milk shake and making it easier to suck out of the cup. PS is no different; the more we add the easier it will be for the patient to take a triggered spontaneous breath. Another point about PS that we need to address again is that the changes need to be small. Your starting point should always be 10 cmH_2O, but any changes up or down need only be by 1 cmH_2O at a time. 1 cmH_2O will equal 75-150 mL of augmented ability in V_t. So you can see that the PS is very sensitive and we do not want our patients using too much. Remember, we want our patients taking some spontaneous breaths, but we do not want them to overwork. Maintaining a maximum of 75% of the targeted V_t based on their IBW is the key. If they were exceeding this during spontaneous breaths, then you would increase their pain and sedation and decrease their PS by 1 cmH$_2$O. Re-evaluation is key and should be looked at closely throughout the patient's transport.

The additional characteristics that SIMV has over AC are very optimal for the transport environment. Just the additional safety aspect of having a mode of ventilation that allows the patient to take a spontaneous breath rather than a full control breath is a big deal. Vibration and movement of the ventilator is a major concern in transport. I have demonstrated this in videos we have released on YouTube where I simply move the ventilator gently back and forth with a trigger setting on 1-2 and the (f) of breaths increase within 10 seconds to 28 breaths per minute. Now imagine if the mode was set to AC and this was happening over a 30-minute flight. It is because of this that SIMV limits any potential hyperventilation or breath stacking and is more comfortable for the patient.

Despite the great aspects of PS and augmented spontaneous breaths, SIMV can also cause some potential issues. If you allow the patient too much effort, it may lead to respiratory fatigue and be counter-productive for patients that are already in respiratory compromise. Because of this, your strategy should be to limit any spontaneous breath to 75% maximum of your set V_t based on their IBW. That means that any spontaneous breath of

300mL would be the maximum for a patient having an IBW calculated V_t of 400mL. Are you thinking…how can we identify the amount of their spontaneous breath? That is a great thought. You are limited in this measurement based on the ventilator you are using. The LTV1200, ReVel and Hamilton T1 ventilators all give the clinician the spontaneous exhaled tidal volume. My strategy on these patients is to not worry so much about their overall volume, but always make sure that I am treating the patient's pain and sedation adequately. I want the patient to take a few spontaneous breaths, but do not want them to overwork at the same time. Because of this, I will look at the overall (f) on the settings screen, which represents the set respiratory rate and spontaneously triggered breaths. If my set rate is 18 and am now seeing (f) of 28 per minute, I know that my pain and sedation status may need addressing.

I would be remiss to not mention a potential issue with SIMV. You can have a potential phenomenon called ventilator asynchrony. Because the mode of ventilation allows our patients the benefit of taking trigger generated spontaneous breaths, the ventilator has to synchronize itself so as to not deliver a control breath during or right after the triggered breath. This aspect of SIMV is one of its primary functions as stated in its name – "**synchronized** intermittent mandatory ventilation". It is meant to synchronize and time spontaneous breaths with control breaths, however ventilator-patient asynchrony may occur. If this does happen, you can do a manual breath and/or give the patient more sedation. More often than not, the reason this occurs is due to too many triggered breaths being taken by the patient.

One of the biggest misconceptions with SIMV is that it is used so that patients do not have respiratory muscle atrophy. Although studies have shown that patients come off the ventilator quicker if weaning can be achieved quicker, respiratory muscles do not atrophy. If you think about this statement it is a little comical. Our respiratory muscles are essentially our diaphragms. Our diaphragm is innervated and fired via our phrenic nerve located in our spinal cord. Unless we have a high cervical spine injury between C3-C5, our diaphragm will continue to fire until we die. Obviously there are other disease processes that can cause diaphragmatic paralysis, but for the illustration of modes of ventilation and the argument for and against one mode vs. another, this just does not pan out. In the end, it is your judgment and opinion on what mode you want to use. It comes down to critical thinking and identifying your settings and what is going to benefit your patient the most.

Continuous Positive Airway Pressure (CPAP)

Continuous positive airway pressure (CPAP) is a great tool that we started using in the EMS and HEMS industry about 15 years ago. Over time, it has been shown to be very beneficial for multiple patient presentations including COPD, asthma, CHF and general respiratory failure. For patients with COPD and asthma, CPAP overpowers the residual pressure that prevents the lungs from fully emptying on exhalation. This decreases the patient's workload and increases oxygenation. Essentially CPAP = PEEP = EPAP. This means that they are the same thing as far as the physiology involved with maintaining alveolar patency.

In the pediatric population, positive intrapulmonary pressure is applied artificially to the airways, whereby distending pressure is created in the alveoli throughout the respiratory cycle in a spontaneously breathing baby. It prevents alveolar atelectasis and enhances and maintains functional residual capacity (FRC) resulting in reopening of collapsed/unstable alveoli leading to improved oxygenation and ventilation.

Many times CPAP or BiPAP (we will discuss this in the next section) can be applied and prevent intubation all together. I do not think we utilize these delivery methods enough and should be training on the potential benefits on a consistent basis. As much as we all like intubation, treating respiratory failure or decompensation can be achieved using CPAP or BiPAP, which decreases ventilator-associated problems including ventilator-associated pneumonia, delirium and longer ICU stays.

CPAP is applied using the ventilator and initiating the CPAP mode. Once this is applied, you are accessing the EPAP (which is the PEEP button on the ventilator) and placing a starting EPAP most often at 10 cmH$_2$O. This will change based on the patient and different scenarios related to size and age. Honestly, CPAP is not used as much as BiPAP due to BiPAP's ability to deliver pressure in a bi-level manner. This is more comfortable for the patient and aids in CO_2 off-loading due to the patient's ability to exhale over a lower pressure level.

Benefits:

- Increases the functional residual capacity (FRC)
- Decreases shunt and opens collapsed alveoli
- Reduces the work of breathing by improving atelectasis and V/Q ratio
- Effective for treatment of pulmonary edema, CHF, COPD and asthma
- Reduces preload and afterload
- Improves oxygenation and hypercapnia

Bi-Level Positive Airway Pressure (BiPAP)

In contrast to CPAP, bi-level positive airway pressure (BiPAP) can be described as a continuous positive airway pressure system with a time-cycled or flow-cycled change of the applied CPAP level by using PEEP. It delivers a preset inspiratory positive airway pressure (IPAP) and expiratory positive airway pressure (EPAP) by applying PEEP. This mode of delivery is better overall and is used more consistently in treating patients. Let's look at how to apply BiPAP in different patient presentations.

For patients with predominantly hypoxemic respiratory failure, start with the recommended initial BiPAP settings. If the expected response, increase in oxygenation, is not achieved, increase the EPAP in increments of 2 cmH_2O with each adjustment. But, keep the gradient between IPAP and EPAP the same, such that the IPAP will be increased by the same increments as the EPAP.

In situations of predominately hypercapnic respiratory

failure, the goal is to improve the tidal volume and the minute ventilation. Settings may be initiated with a wider gradient between IPAP and EPAP. If the expected response, a decrease in carbon dioxide, is not achieved, increase the gradient between IPAP and EPAP.

Remember that most often it is a mixed respiratory failure. So we may start with IPAP of 10 over EPAP of 5. If the oxygenation is not acceptable, attempt to improve the oxygenation. Increase the IPAP and EPAP, but keep the gradient the same. If the ventilation is not optimal, the settings need to be adjusted to increase the tidal volume. This is achieved with an increase in the gradient between IPAP and EPAP.

For hypoxemic respiratory failure, keep the gradient the same and increase both the IPAP and EPAP. For hypercapnic respiratory failure, widen the gradient between them so as to have the EPAP lower, which allows for easier exhalation and exhalation pressures.

Last, one of the big concerns when flying patients on BiPAP is the consumption of oxygen. Unless your aircraft is equipped with liquid oxygen, you better make sure you have a full main tank with an extra pony bottle. One way to conserve oxygen in these patients is to utilize a feature found on the LTV1000 and 1200 called O2 conserve. While the ReVel ventilator does not have an O_2 conserve feature, it allows you to turn down the bias flow to 3L/min. So what is O_2 conserve? It is the way to turn off the bias-flow. Remember the bias-flow is the flow through the circuit during exhalation. This is how most ventilators are triggered (flow triggered). During BiPAP, in most cases there is no need to have the bias-flow active during the exhalation process (EPAP). How do we activate this? This is activated in the ventilator menu settings screen under "Ventilator Control". When you turn this on it will only deliver (flow) FiO_2 during the IPAP phase of BiPAP. During the exhalation phase or EPAP, the (flow) FiO_2 will be cut off. This significantly reduces oxygen consumption and will benefit you and your patient!

Based on my above explanation, there are a few very important things to point out regarding your IPAP and EPAP. Depending on the type device you are using for BiPAP; either a stand-alone machine or a mechanical ventilator, your IPAP and EPAP ratio are different. Based on that statement, there are two terms we need to understand.

Additive – Ventilators are said to be additive or "PEEP Compensated". This means that the PS is in addition to the PEEP or better said, IPAP is in addition to EPAP. Simply said – PEEP compensated.

Absolute – Stand-alone are said to be absolute. This means that the IPAP and EPAP are separate and not in addition to each other. Simply said – not PEEP compensated.

Now that we understand this difference, how does this look on our ventilators? If you were told by a physician that your patient needs to be initially set at an IPAP of 12 and EPAP of 5, and are using a mechanical ventilator like the LTV 1200 or Revel for example, you would need to remember the term "Additive". This means that your IPAP is in addition to your PEEP (EPAP). So you would want your (PS) IPAP set at 7 cmH$_2$O and (PEEP) EPAP set at 5 cmH$_2$O (IPAP 7 + EPAP 5 = IPAP 12). This would then give you an IPAP of 12 and EPAP of 5. You will also see this reflected in your PIP. Your PIP will read no less than your IPAP over EPAP number. For the above example this would be a PIP of 12.

This is a very important concept to understand and will really help reduce high pressures that are counter-productive for overall ventilation (IPAP). Often times exceeding an IPAP of 20 cmH$_2$O will lead to increased mask leaks, gastric inflation and increased patient anxiety. In addition, PIP > 30 cmH$_2$O (IPAP + EPAP) will also lead to gastric inflation and a potential risk for vomiting and aspiration.

Chapter 4 – Advanced Modes of Ventilation

Pressure Regulated Volume Control (PRVC)

As we have discussed in the section above on pressure ventilation, this mode of delivery has been shown to be the safest and most optimal for those sick "baby" lungs. Pressure regulated volume control (PRVC) is an excellent mode of ventilation that is used predominantly in the hospital setting now days. It is also the additional mode of ventilation that the new ReVel and Hamilton T1 ventilators have available. One of the biggest attributes this mode encompasses is the ability to improve oxygenation due to constant pressure and decreased inspiratory flow patterns. The ventilator adjusts pressure based on the patient's airway resistance and respiratory system compliance changes in order to deliver the set tidal volume. The ventilator monitors each breath for V_t. If the delivered V_t is too low, it increases the inspiratory pressure on the next breath. If it is too high, it decreases the pressure. It measures this by examining the V_{te} and compares it to the desired V_t.

See the table and ventilator algorithm below for a better illustration of how the mode works.

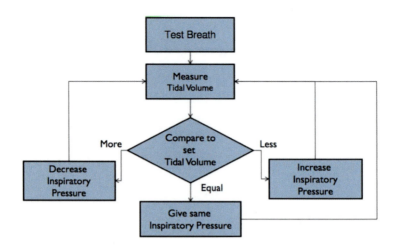

The PRVC mode of ventilation set-up is just the same as all modes. You will identify your IBW, V_t, RR, PEEP, I:E ratio and FiO_2. The ventilator will now do some cool things. PRVC is considered a duel mode of delivery for a few reasons. First, the ventilator starts out in volume. You have already set your Vt and standard settings. From there, the ventilator identifies the starting inspiratory pressure (PEEP + 10), then uses that calculation to switch to pressure. It uses that reading to initiate pressure delivery. If the PEEP was 5 cmH_2O, then it will start with 15 cmH_2O as the inspiratory pressure and target the tidal volume you have pre-set in the ventilator. It then compares the delivered pressure breath exhaled tidal volume (V_{te}) with the pre-set V_t and then adjusts the pressure up if the V_{te} was lower than the pre-set V_t or lowers the pressure if the Vte was higher than the pre-set V_t. With that in mind, we need to understand pressure maximums. We never want our pressure to exceed 35 cmH_2O. That is the middle point between our high P_{plat} (30 cmH_2O) range and our high PIP (40 cmH_2O) range. This will prevent the regulated pressure from increasing higher and higher in an attempt to achieve the pre-set V_t we have set in the ventilator. If our patient started having issues with air-trapping and auto-PEEP, and chest compliance started decreasing, the ventilator would not be able to achieve the same V_t based on the same pressure. As such, the PRVC mode would continue to increase the inspiratory pressure in an attempt to achieve that V_t. Setting the upper pressure limit of 35 cmH$_2$O will limit that risk of high pressure, however will not limit the risk for decompensation. The teaching point here is that the upper pressure limit may stop the ventilator from increasing to high levels that may cause injury, but will not stop the issues associated with air-trapping, auto-PEEP or decreasing chest compliance. Always continue to assess the Vte and trend this number consistently when using pressure ventilation modes so you can identify any of these trends.

Now that we have discussed the characteristics of the mode, let's discuss a few things about the mode as it relates to the transport environment. Because the mode is called the "learning" or "smart" mode of ventilation and its primary function is to regulate the pressure in the hopes of targeting your pre-set V_t, it is then dependent on consistency. What I mean by this is it is all about the trigger and any interruptions seen with the ventilator. Basically if the ventilator has any type of change made (RR, I-time, PEEP), interruption, or is disconnected, then it will take 5-6 breaths to re-learn the regulation pressure. With that being said, PRVC has many great attributes, but may be a better mode for hospital patients vs. transport patients. My experience has been positive, however the concerns about pressure regulation problems due to changes made to the ventilator, interruptions or disconnections could be counterproductive for patients needing consistent ventilatory support. Great care should be taken if used in the transport environment to limit these issues and maintain consistent ventilator support.

Adaptive Support Ventilation (ASV)

Adaptive support ventilation (ASV) is a mode of ventilation found in the transport environment, specifically on the Hamilton T1 ventilator. This mode of ventilation is a microprocessor-controlled mode of mechanical ventilation that provides an automatic selection of continuous breath-by-breath adaptation of the RR and V_t. The clinician inputs whether the patient is male or female and an estimated height. The ventilator then identifies, based on IBW, the desired VE for that patient. As such, the clinician does not have any control over the set RR or V_t while using this mode. Why? Because ASV uses a concept called the "Otis" least work of breathing formula to determine the RR and V_t. This is why it is called "adaptive".

Now let's discuss the application of ASV. One of the selling points for ASV is that it is "hands off". The mode takes care of everything and the clinician does not need to worry about anything. This is a very dangerous mindset to have and I would caution you in this way of thinking. One issue that often happens with this mode is how the RR and V_t are delivered. We know that the ventilator has identified a VE per IBW. It then delivers the RR and V_t to achieve the identified VE from your initial IBW input based on the patient's height. One thing the mode will do is never sacrifice V_t for RR. That being said, it may drop the RR and increase $V_t > 8$ mL/kg. An observational study by Dongelmans et al., (May 2011), showed that patients moved from PCV to ASV had a significant reduction in RR and corresponding increase is V_t in patients with ALI. Interestingly, patients that had less compliant lungs (more injured), ASV maintained $V_t < 8$ mL/kg. In contrast, with patients having more compliant lungs (less injured), ASV delivered $V_t > 8$ mL/kg. This was corrected by way of a pressure limit, but your patient's VE will drop to unacceptable ranges. The authors concluded that ASV delivered possible unsafe RR-V_t combinations in patients with ALI and being ventilated using an open lung concept.

Now obviously, this is one study, with a small sample size. The important thing to remember is to always know what your ventilator is doing. Do not take the standpoint of "ASV will do it for me"! You are the one that is trained and should understand what is happening with your ventilator at all times.

Airway Pressure Release Ventilation (APRV)

Airway Pressure Release Ventilation is a mode of ventilation that is specific to only a few transport ventilators on the market today. The most common one is the Hamilton T1. This mode of ventilation uses the concept of high mean airway pressures (MAP) for severely hypoxic patients. This is a common mode for refractory hypoxic patients in acute respiratory distress syndrome (ARDS) and other lung pathophysiologies that need high airway pressures and alveolar recruitment to maintain adequate oxygenation. The APRV mode is a form of bi-level ventilation but utilizes very short expiratory times for pressure release. Think of APRV as a mode like CPAP that uses inverse I:E ratios to provide long inspiratory phases (T_{high}) of 4-6 seconds and short expiratory phases (T_{low}) or "pressure release" of 0.4-0.6 seconds. This delivery is all about optimizing oxygenation and transalveolar pressures and less on PCO_2 levels. Obviously these patients will become more hypercapnic, but remember we live better on the hypercapnic than hypocapnic side.

Often, when establishing APRV, you are actually moving your patient from other starting modes like PRVC or PCV. When moving the patient to APRV because of refractory hypoxia, the starting high PEEP level will be set at the mean airway pressure (MAP) from the previous mode. If starting with APRV as your initial mode, start your high PEEP at 28-30 cmH_2O and work your way down. This translates to higher transalveolar pressures that result in better alveolar recruitment. Once the high PEEP P_{high} is set, you need to set your low PEEP. The low PEEP P_{low} is set at (0 cmH_2O). The larger pressure ramp allows for tidal ventilation in very short expiratory time settings as I have stated above (0.4-0.6 seconds).

Another great tip to remember is based on having high PEEP (CPAP) of >30 cmH_2O. In this setting the spontaneous breaths can have augmentation help via pressure support (PS). However, the P_{plat} should not exceed 30 cmH_2O. This leads to lower Pplat pressures, decreased sedation and near elimination of long-acting paralysis.

Lastly, mean airway pressure (MAP) is everything when attempting to fix refractory hypoxic patients with severe diffusion shunts. Based on this, MAP >12 cmH$_2$O are a must; and the standard, or "norm", we discussed in the section on mean airway pressure cannot be utilized. These patients need these high pressures and any corresponding reduction seen in hemodynamic status should be augmented with vasopressors like norepinephrine, vasopressin and epinephrine drips.

In the end, APRV is a mode that is much more advanced than standard modes often employed in the standard transport environment. The most common clinical setting for this mode to be utilized is the highly acute ARDS patients and in the neonatal population with associated hyaline membrane disease (*neonatal ARDS*), pulmonary hypoplasia (*arrested development of the lungs, alveoli and distal airways*) and refractory hypoxia secondary to under-developed lungs and reduced surfactant levels because of prematurity in early birth situations. However, a recent review of literature by Mireles-Cabodevila and Kacmarek (June 2016), showed no benefit in patient outcomes when using APRV over inverse I:E ratio and SIMV-PC, with the final conclusion based on the literature review showing a greater potential for adverse outcomes.

High Frequency Ventilation (HFV)

High frequency ventilation is a mode of ventilation that is focused on primarily the neonate and pediatric population. The goal of HFV is to maintain the highest amount of alveolar recruitment with the smallest tidal volumes possible so as to not add to any barotrauma potential, while at the same time allowing preservation of end expiratory lung volume to minimize barotrauma. This is accomplished by providing the tidal volume at a level at or below the dead space volume and then delivering them at a supraphysiologic frequency.

Although HFV is used as a stand-alone mode of high frequency ventilation, most high frequency ventilators use either high frequency oscillatory ventilation (HFOV) or high frequency jet ventilation (HFJV). We will explore both of those modes of delivery in the sections below.

High Frequency Oscillatory Ventilation (HFOV)

High frequency oscillatory ventilation (HFOV) is a mode of ventilation that is primarily used in the pediatric and neonatal population. This manner of delivery is said to be more unconventional in comparison to standard modes of ventilation, with the goal focusing on maintaining lung recruitment and avoiding barotrauma. HFOV uses techniques to maintain the most optimal alveolar recruitment by delivering mean airway pressures that are much higher than what is perceived as normal. This means that the peak inspiratory pressure (PIP) may be higher than the normal high (>40 cmH$_2$O), that we evaluate for our standard modes of ventilation. However, the ventilations are delivered in a much different manner than our conventional modes of delivery. HFOV instead provides ventilations through piston driven sinusoidal pressure oscillations (ΔP) at a frequency between 3 – 15 hertz. The goal of the oscillatory pressure (ΔP) is to produce visible chest vibration from the level of the clavicles to the lower abdomen or pelvis.

So how is this mode determined or initiated for our patients. Again, this mode of ventilation is very specific and used in most cases with neonatal and pediatric patients with a high risk for barotrauma, pulmonary hypoplasia, hyaline membrane disease, mean airway pressures that are exceeding 18-20 cmH$_2$O, ALI, and ARDS. Remember that our ideal mean airway pressure (MAP) should normally be <12 cmH$_2$O. As discussed in the section on MAP, often times modes of ventilation that focus on delivering high MAPs in an attempt to recruit alveoli in patients with refractory hypoxia or atelectasis trauma will utilize a MAP > 12 cmH$_2$O. If you identify your patient would be a candidate for HFOV, your patient will be suffering from high peak inspiratory pressures (PIP). The starting PIP will be set via HFOV at 3-5 cmH$_2$O above the PIP on the conventional mode of ventilation you were using immediately prior to transition to HFOV. After placement on the new mode, your focus should be on optimizing oxygenation by increasing the PIP in 1-2 cmH$_2$O increments until you see an improvement in the oxygenation status. This will then allow you to titrate the FiO2 below the recommended 0.60 or 60%. Your additional focus will be to evaluate lung expansion and overall recruitment by evaluating the patient's chest x-ray and evaluating that both hemidiaphragms project at the level of the 8th to 10th posterior rib.

How do you evaluate your ventilation? Your evaluation focuses on the amplitude oscillatory pressure, by increasing the (ΔP) in 2-3 cmH$_2$O increments in an attempt to improve CO2 clearance. The total amount of chest wiggle is fluctuated by adjusting the amount of delta P (PIP – PEEP) on the ventilator. In addition to changes in the oscillatory pressure (ΔP), you can influence the ventilation by adjusting the frequency. The amount of frequency is inversely related to the tidal volume in the mode of delivery. That means that the high frequencies will generally deliver tidal volumes of 1-3 mL/kg.

High Frequency Jet Ventilation

High frequency jet ventilation is a mode of ventilation that utilizes a jet injector near the level of the carina at a very high velocity. To achieve this type of delivery, a special endotracheal tube (ETT) with a jet injector is utilized to augment this form of mechanical ventilation. If the transport team does not have this special ETT, or if a special ETT is not available at the referring facility, an in-line jet injector adaptor is added to the existing ETT. The goal of this mode of delivery is to provide respiratory rates at 100 to 600 bpm at a V_t of 3-5 mL/kg.

One of the biggest risks to this manner of delivery is based on the jet injector and potential injury to the airway at or near the level of the carina. There is also a high risk for air trapping with these patients, so great care should be taken to evaluate compliance in an ongoing manner. As I stated above, the most common form of HFV is that of HFOV, with HFJV being used in pediatrics that are < 8 years of age due to the limitation in delivering minute ventilations that are high enough for patients above that age demographic.

Helium-Oxygen (Heliox)

As we discussed in previous sections, gases have characteristics that make them small and light, which allows them to diffuse easier, or in contrast gases are heavy and more dense in nature, and have poor diffusion capabilities. Heliox is a biologically inert gas that has a very low density in comparison to nitrogen and oxygen. This means that the molecules are very small and light. This allows the gas to diffuse very quickly and rapidly.

Helium is added to oxygen and forms Heliox, with a mixture of 80:20 or 70:30 respectively. It is important to always utilize a helium-oxygen mixture and never utilize pure helium alone; always administer with oxygen! With inhalation, the resistance to airflow is then reduced (small molecules) and the areas of turbulent flow through obstructed airways are converted to a more streamline non-turbulent flow, thereby improving the patient's work of breathing.

Why would we ever use Heliox? What disease processes would benefit? The most common patients that would benefit from this type of gas mixture would be those that are classified as obstructive lung patients. This subgroup of patients has underlying pathophysiologies of asthma, stridor, croup, bronchopulmonary dysplasia and overall high airway resistance. By using the Heliox mixture, oxygen can then penetrate those distal airways much easier due to the small molecular make up of helium. Airways that otherwise would not get therapy now will be reached due to the added ability of the helium molecule to reach the most distal obstructive airways. This treatment is widely used in the administration of bronchodilator medications for patients with severe obstruction airflow diseases. This therapy allows time for onset of therapeutic medications or the resolution of the disease process. If this therapy is successful it may prevent intubation, with the benefits of the Heliox administration evident within several minutes.

Nitric Oxide (iNO)

We have all become aware of nitric oxide's ability in our lungs to cause selective vasodilation without causing systemic hypotension. We see nitric oxide's benefit during its diffusion across the alveolar capillary membrane, with the smooth muscle cells in the adjacent pulmonary vessels relaxing as a result. This in-turn causes a lower pulmonary vasculature resistance (PVR). As discussed in sections previous to this one, the ability to maintain the perfect V/Q match is our body's goal in homeostasis. Oxygenation increases as the iNO diffuses across the alveolar-capillary membrane, thus redistributing blood flow and reducing intrapulmonary shunting,

When would it be the most optimal to utilize this form of therapy? Based on nitric oxide's mechanism of action, patients that suffer from pulmonary hypertension and isolated right heart failure benefit greatly from iNO therapy. As such, we see this used extensively in the neonatal-pediatric population.

Before we jump into this pathophysiology, let's first remember how fetal circulation is different while the fetus is in utero. Because right-sided heart pressures are higher than left side (PVR > SVR), most of the blood in the right atrium moves to the right ventricle via the foramen ovale. The blood then pushes up into the pulmonary artery. Because we have low oxygen, we see pulmonary arteries that are closed. The blood cannot go through the pulmonary artery and into the lungs and as such the blood moves through the ductus arteriosus and through the body. This is okay because the placenta already oxygenates the blood. In this setting, the neonate's heart is said to have a high-pressure right side and low pressure left side. This is much different than after the neonate is born, with their heart moving to a low pressure right side and high pressure left side. This is where the issues start, regarding heart defects and our topic of pulmonary hypertension.

Neonates that suffer from acyanotic heart defects like neonatal CHF, ventral septal defect (VSD), tetralogy of fallot and pulmonary artery obstruction defects, have secondary pulmonary hypertension. Why does this happen? Pulmonary hypertension is caused as a result of prolonged hypoxia. The pulmonary vasculature constricts to keep oxygenated blood in the lungs. This results in profound hypertension. PVR > SVR, meaning the right atrium becomes the higher pressure compared to the left atrium. Blood shunts from right to left causing un-oxygenated blood moving to the systemic system leading to profound hypoxia. One therapy that is added to help reduce the pulmonary hypertension is focused on keeping the neonate on the alkalotic side, with the pH goal being 7.45-7.55. This in-turn relieves some of the pulmonary hypertension by causing vasodilation.

Administration of iNO can be done via a nasal cannula or ventilator circuit. Remember that any neonate or pediatric patient will benefit from a simple nasal cannula with or without iNO due to the nasal cannulas ability to apply PEEP in these patients. The dose range is between 5 to 40 ppm (parts per million). An important treatment pearl to remember with administration is focused on never abruptly stopping iNO therapy without consultation from the receiving or referring physician. Doing so will cause pulmonary vascular resistance (PVR) to increase significantly and cause acute hypoxia and right ventricular dysfunction as a result. Lastly, it is also very important to evaluate any alveolar cytotoxicity related to methemoglobinemia. This is a rare complication with iNO administration, but one that needs to be evaluated via ABG analysis through the care of your patients.

Chapter 5 – Ventilator Strategy

Acute Lung Injury (ALI) and ARDS

Acute lung injury (ALI) and ARDS is a big issue facing millions of patients we may transport. What is ALI and how does this manifest into other, more traditional disease processes?

Despite the initial injury or illness, anyone is potentially a candidate for what is called an inflammatory response. This happens for multiple reasons that include the injury or illness itself, fluid administration, or barotrauma from over-ventilation.

The inflammatory response manifests itself by releasing inflammatory mediators that promote neutrophil accumulation in the microcirculation. These mediators cause vascular permeability and gaps in the alveolar-capillary epithelial membrane, which leads to pulmonary edema and loss of surfactant.

In the early stages, increased permeability of the alveolar-capillary membrane causes an influx of fluid into the alveoli, which causes interstitial fluid build-up. This results in breakdown and actually causes the alveoli to separate from the capillaries.

The later stage is called the fibroproliferative phase, which causes an infiltration of fibroblasts that lead to collagen deposition, fibrosis and worsening hypoxic respiratory failure. Finally, as a protective mechanism, the patient will have pulmonary vasoconstriction, which leads to more fluid into the interstitial spaces. This further separates the alveolar-capillary membrane and makes it even harder to oxygenate them at this point.

Diagnostic criteria to identify ALI vs. ARDS:

- **Chest x-ray will show bilateral pulmonary infiltrates**
- **Pulmonary capillary wedge pressure <18 mmHg**
- **PaO_2/FiO_2 <300 = ALI**
- **PaO_2/FiO_2 <200 = ARDS**

1. *ARDS must be differentiated from pneumonia or CHF. CHF is characterized by fluid overload, whereas patients with ARDS do not show signs of left atrial HTN or overt volume overload.*
2. *Wedge pressure (8-12 mmHg) is a reflection of LVEDP; so if the wedge is high, it is probably not ARDS but pulmonary edema from a cardiogenic source.*
3. *The severity of hypoxemia is necessary to make the diagnosis. This is defined by the ratio of the partial pressure of oxygen in the patient's arterial blood to the fraction of O_2 in the inspired air.*

4. *If <300, then it is ALI (they may be getting ARDS, but not sick enough to be considered ARDS yet). If <200, this is indicative of ARDS.*

As you can see this disease process is horrible and is estimated that 7% of all patients admitted to the ICU and 16% of patients on mechanical ventilation will develop ALI or ARDS. Most ARDS-related deaths are due to multi-organ failure. However in children, ARDS is much less common and less likely to lead to death.

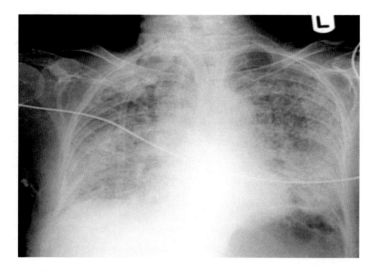

If you look closely at the above chest x-ray, you will see diffuse bilateral infiltrates that are often seen as gravity dependent. You will also notice an appearance often referred to as "ground glass". These are patchy opacities noted throughout the lung fields. (This resembles taking a cotton ball and dabbing it throughout the lung fields). Associated bilateral pleural effusions can occur in 50% of patients as well. It is sometimes difficult to distinguish between ARDS and pulmonary edema. If the patient were given Lasix,

Improvement would be noted if the patient had pulmonary edema but would not improve if ARDS were present.

Treatment options:

The only way to improve the patient is to oxygenate and ventilate them so they can heal themselves and the alveoli can become healthy again. Because ARDS causes an increase in intrapulmonary shunting and severe hypoxemia, a higher FiO_2 is normally required to maintain adequate tissue oxygenation and lung recruitment with PEEP. However, care should be taken to optimize oxygenation status with the lowest FiO_2 possible. Higher PEEP levels accomplish this. Lung protective strategies should be initiated at 4-6 mL/kg.

ARDS Network Study

As you can see from the above section on ALI and ARDS, this disease process is responsible for taking millions of lives around the world each year. Based on this, the National Heart, Lung, and Blood Institute and National Institute of Health established a clinical network to carry out multi-center clinical trials of ARDS treatment (ARDS Network, par. 1). The main goal of the ARDS network is to test potential treatment theories, agents, devices and new strategies to improve the overall care and survival rates among patients suffering from ARDS.

I wanted to cite some of the relevant material based on the work done by the ARDS Network group. If you look at ARDS and the historically high mortality rates, the relevant studies this group has completed have been groundbreaking. As such, we now use lung protective strategies for our ventilator dependent patients and have seen improved survival, shortened duration of mechanical ventilation and associated conservative fluid management.

The most important lessons learned from these studies have been the lung protective strategies. We now use this strategy for all ventilator dependent patients in an attempt to treat ARDS and ALI. In addition, conservative use of fluid administration, combined with excess fluid removal by using diuretics, have lessened the need for mechanical ventilation and reduced overall ICU stays. With that being said, the ARDS Network researchers have established groundbreaking strategies that have saved lives. However, despite these strategies, severe cases of ARDS still have a 40 percent mortality rate (ARDS Network par. 5). Despite this, we should applaud their work and employ the lung protective strategies on all of our ventilator dependent patients.

The Injury Approach

Now that we have made it this far in the book, let's now focus on the strategy behind mechanical ventilation. I think the most frustrating aspect of mechanical ventilation for many clinicians is not understanding how to approach different patients. With that being said, there is an excellent way to do this. Simply divide your patients into two categories. Having just two different strategies will allow you to focus these clinical strategies to your mechanically ventilated patients. The two different strategies are the injury and obstructive strategies. Essentially there are two patient presentations that encompass the obstructive strategy – COPD and asthma. Every other patient presentation will fall under the injury strategy. It is that simple! These strategies will focus on specific features that add protection to your patients and optimize your treatment strategies for their overall disease process.

The injury approach to ventilation is simple: focus on protecting the patient's lungs from further harm. If you think about the patients we transport, you could argue that most of them have some type of sick or injured "baby" lung. I use the baby lung analogy because we need to understand the magnitude of how potentially harmful our treatments may be to these patients. As we have discussed in sections above, many patients suffer from ALI and then ARDS. Many times a simple disease process leads to inflammatory responses alone, but mismanagement of our ventilator strategies also play a large role in ALI. It is because of this that the protection for the injury approach is low Vt and higher rates. The goal is to maintain minute ventilations that allow for lung protection, but still optimize eucapnia and proper gas exchange goals. Your underlying mode of ventilation does not change, as SIMV + PS will be my choice 9 times out of 10. Your V_t range will be 4-6 mL/kg and your respiratory rates will be based on the formulas we learned in chapter 2 of 100 mL/kg/min for VE. If you remember that would give you a rate of 16 breaths per minute. If you are thinking to yourself, geez that is a high rate, you are correct. But if you think about maintaining minute ventilation that adds protection for those sick "baby" lungs, our goals have to be centered on a low Vt and higher rates to achieve alveolar minute ventilation that aids in gas exchange, but still protects those sick lungs. In addition, remember the amount of volume we lose in dead space and it should make sense that a higher rate is needed. In addition to watching your V_t, it is also important to trend your patients P_{plat} often and then attempt to reduce this if >30 cmH$_2$O using the strategies we discussed in chapter 2.

Lastly, your strategies that involve I-time, I:E ratio and FiO$_2$ will also be based on our discussions in chapter 2. I think the biggest thing to consider is your FiO$_2$ and the strategies involved with the patient's current presentation and pathophysiology. In the acute phase of any illness, it is okay to give as much FiO$_2$ as needed, but always consider all aspects of your patient's clinical situation; including Hgb, Hct, SvO$_2$, ABG, and Do$_2$ if available.

The Obstructive Approach

Not unlike the injury approach to ventilation, the obstructive approach is all about protection. If you think about obstructive lung patients, the biggest factor for these patients is the inability to exhale properly. As we discussed in sections earlier, maintaining good ventilation (removal and regulation of CO$_2$) is the biggest factor seen in overall ventilator management. You couple that with a patient that has a disease process that limits this even further and you have a nightmare waiting to manifest.

Based on the patient's pathophysiology of narrowed and brittle airways, obstructive lung patients just cannot get the air back out. It is because of this simple but forgotten factor that the entire protective strategy for the obstructive approach is centered on reduction of the respiratory rate. If you consider a few factors regarding hypoxia, and our response to hypoxia, it will make sense in how these patients decompensate so quickly. When we become hypoxic or have any type of sympathetic response, we increase our respiratory rate. COPD and asthma patients do the same thing. As such, they become hypoxic, then tachypneic, which causes a reduction in expiratory time. They are spending the entire time inhaling due to the high respiratory rate and never given enough time to exhale. Once they start the exhalation process they take another breath and this starts that rapid phenomenon called air-trapping and auto-PEEP. Remember that we only have so much time to inhale and exhale. This causes these patients to continue to decompensate quickly. As their air-trapping and auto-PEEP increase, this causes worsening chest compliance and they are now attempting to breathe over those excessive pressures. These patients already have weak chest wall muscles and fatigue quickly.

The strategy is to give a V_t in the 6-8 mL/kg range and then limit the respiratory rate to 10-12 breaths per minute. In many of these patients, starting V_t will most often be on the higher end of our range, with 8 mL/kg being most optimal. Any associated hypoxia will slowly resolve based on your ability to decrease the air-trapping and improve compliance. Often, the hypoxia is a result of a low V_t secondary to poor chest wall compliance from the air-trapping phenomenon. In addition to employing this strategy, it is important to optimize the exhalation time as well by adjusting the I-time and I:E ratio. A reduction in I-time should be focused on an I:E ratio of 1:4.1-1:6.1 in severe cases. In addition, pharmacological treatments should be focused on beta-2 agonists, anticholinergic agents and steroid therapy.

Another controversial topic in obstructive lung patients is the use of PEEP or lack thereof. We need to understand a few things about auto-PEEP and its significance on lung compliance and hemodynamics. Patients that suffer from COPD and asthma often live with an auto-PEEP phenomenon. We need to remember that these patients have this presentation normally, although not in excess, and we will not be able to or should not expect to reduce their auto-PEEP to physiological norms of 3-5 cmH_2O. With that being said, most patients in obstructive respiratory failure will benefit from PEEP of 3-5 cmH_2O. We need to remember that PEEP aids in maintaining alveolar recruitment during the exhalation process. These patients have diseased alveolar sacs and will benefit from some PEEP. Atelectasis trauma is a common issue and without PEEP, these patients will not have optimal recruitment.

Let me explain this in another way. Our obstructive lung patients have airflow obstruction. External PEEP is employed to decrease the work of breathing and is not a treatment for the underlying condition. Many clinicians have argued that adding PEEP to these patients will worsen the auto-peep phenomenon.

According to the 2005 article by Mughal et al.:

This can be explained with the following analogy regarding a stream with a waterfall. In this analogy, the upstream part of the stream is like the distal airways, the downstream part of the stream is like the proximal airways, and the waterfall is like the site of critical airway closure. Pressure in the airways is like the hydrostatic pressure in the stream. Now suppose the tide comes in (external PEEP is applied), raising the height of the stream below the waterfall. This has no effect on either the flow or the pressure upstream of the waterfall unless the water level rises above the level of the waterfall (if the level of external PEEP exceeds the critical closing pressure). Above this level, external PEEP increases the pressure upstream and exacerbates hyperinflation. However, if external PEEP is kept below 75% to 85% of the auto-PEEP level, worsening hyperinflation or circulatory depression are unlikely to occur (2005).

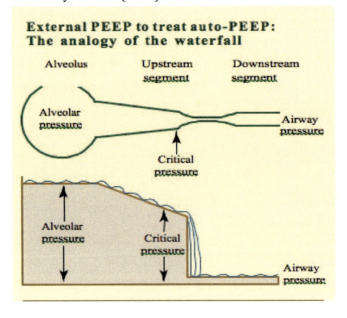

Why does external PEEP help? In patients with auto-PEEP, if the ventilator is set to deliver patient targeted breaths, the inspiratory muscles have to produce an initial effort to overcome the opposing recoil pressure before the ventilator can be triggered and inspiratory flow can begin. In that respect, auto-PEEP acts as an inspiratory threshold and represents additional impedance that the respiratory muscles have to face (Mughal et al., 2005). Adding PEEP in these circumstances, or for that matter BiPAP, will reduce the work of breathing. A practical method of determining whether your patient may benefit from PEEP application is to watch the cycling PIP pressure. If the PIP changes very little when you apply PEEP then these patients will benefit from the PEEP application. On the other hand, if you see an increase in PIP that is based on the PEEP application, this may mean that the PEEP may be causing hyperinflation. With that being said, applying PEEP prophylactically to all patients with an airflow obstruction is not ideal. Only patients with auto-PEEP and flow limitations with associated dynamic airway compression will potentially benefit (Mughal et al., 2005). In addition, we have to remember, when dealing with these patients, that you are employing many different strategies, including lower respiratory rates, extended I:E ratios and pharmacological intervention. Because of this, be careful not to make too many changes at once. You will never know what actually made the patient better. In the end, auto-PEEP is always relevant to the patient's normal levels. We need not be concerned with this unless we see significant hemodynamic compromise that is a result of the auto-PEEP and not some other clinical presentation.

Ventilator Associated Pneumonia (VAP)

I would be remiss if I did not add a section on ventilator-associated pneumonia (VAP). VAP is an infection in patients who have an ETT in place and are ventilator dependent, with pneumonia occurring within 48 hours post-intubation. In the ICU it is the leading cause of acquired illness. It is important that as transport providers we take the necessary steps to aid in the prevention of VAP. In addition, as transport provider crews who perform advance airway management, we should be very familiar with this complication. Deedle (2013) found 20% of the incidences of VAP occurred in ED intubated patients, which were most likely patients intubated in the field. In 2006, 22% of trauma patients intubated in the ED developed VAP.

How does this happen? When patients are intubated or ventilated with a BVM prior to intubation, the potential for VAP starts. We all have secretions in the back of the mouth that accumulate above the bulb of the ETT. This harbors bacteria, which then leak down into the lungs. During BVM ventilations, any secretions and organisms in the mouth are then pushed in the lungs.

The evidence states that the best way to prevent the development of VAP is called a bundle. A bundle is a number of specific nursing actions, when done together, reduce the incidence of ventilator associated events. In the hospital setting, the following things have found to drastically decrease the incidence of VAP.

- **Head of bed elevated**

- **Oral care**
- **Subglottic suctioning**
- **Adequate pain management regimens**
- **Titrated sedation**
- **Daily sedation vacation**
- **Ventilation vacation and weaning trials**
- **Stress ulcer prophylaxis**
- **DVT prophylaxis**

The importance of implementation of these nursing bundles is essential. We have to understand that this is a real threat, with 42% of patients in the ED who stay intubated longer than 48 hours developing VAP. Again, this increases length of stay, ICU days and mortality. We need to be patient advocates in all phases of care.

We can all make a difference by doing a few things and being conscious of prevention strategies.

- *Any ETT with open packages greater than 48 hours need to be disposed of. The literature states organisms grow on the ETT during this time. A best practice is to label the opened package from the date it was opened and then dispose of any ETT after that date.*
- *Limit the attempts with intubations. Make the first attempt the best attempt.*
- *Get the dosage correct with intubations. Stop the use of NO medication intubations. These patients can have a gag reflex and may vomit or aspirate.*
- *Place NGT or OGT on all intubated patients*

Chapter 6 – Alarms

High Pressure Alarms

As we have discussed in chapter 2, your peak inspiratory pressure (PIP) is measured at the peak of inspiration and is a representation of many factors. It includes the volume of each breath, compliance of the lungs, airway resistance and the force needed to deliver the breath. We have learned that your patients PIP needs to be <40 cmH$_2$O. Because of the potential negative effects associated, it is important to set an alarm that will notify the clinician of any high pressure that exceeds those safe zones. As we have discussed, that magic number is 40 cmH$_2$O, however with some patients that may need to be increased based on their current presentation and disease process. An example would be a patient with an inflow obstruction as seen in COPD and asthma. These patients may have PIP significantly greater than 40 cmH$_2$O. It will be your judgment to move the high-pressure alarm up in those cases. We have to remember that we do not want the ventilator alarming throughout the transfer and in those cases turning the alarm up would be warranted.

Low Pressure Alarm

Your low-pressure alarm is also very important. Often times for me this is more important than anything else. This will inform you of any disconnections essentially. If you are reading this book you have probably experienced a ventilator circuit disconnection at some point. Remember to always go through your DOPE pneumonic

(Disconnection, Obstructions, Pneumothorax, Equipment) check anytime you have a low-pressure alarm. Most often this will be due to a circuit disconnection at either the ETT or ventilator connection. In addition, the LTV1000 and 1200 for example, will show a disc-sense error when you have any disconnection. Furthermore, your low-pressure alarm will also activate if you have an O_2 source disconnection or have ran out of oxygen all together. As you can see, this alarm is very important and something that may save your butt.

Low Minute Ventilation Alarm

The low minute ventilation alarm is an excellent warning system for disconnections as well as for patients being ventilated on a pressure initiated manner of delivery. Remember from our discussion in chapter 3, pressure control ventilation is a compliance-based mode. Based on this, your minute ventilation is not guaranteed. Because of the potential changes seen in patient's chest wall compliance, your Vt may change and is always different. The low minute ventilation alarm will inform you of minute ventilations below the point you set in the alarm screen. Our minute ventilation requirements need to be between 4-8L/min, so based on that I often set my alarm at 3 L/min. I feel like this gives me some protection, but still allows some room for fluctuation.

Chapter 7 – Pain and Sedation Management

Fentanyl
- **Narcotic Analgesic**
    - **Dose: 1-2mcg/kg**
    - **Route: IV/IO**
    - **Onset: 1-3 min**
    - **Duration: 15-20 min**
    - **Indications: blunting of circulatory response to intubation or suspected known increased ICP or cardiovascular disease. Continuous pain management for intubated patients.**
    - **Contraindications: allergy to drug components; caution with documented history of rigid chest syndrome**

    * >5mcg/kg to cause respiratory depression *

Pain management in the transport environment is extremely important. Obviously we fly patients that are severely injured and need continued pain assessment and care. Couple this with our ventilated patients and you have patients that are in dire need for continued pain management. We know based on multiple studies that the pain associated with intubation and mechanical ventilation is greater that we could ever imagine. It has been shown to be comparable to second degree burns and the pain associated with cracking someone's chest for heart surgery. With that being said, liberal pain management strategies should always be initiated and continued on all your mechanically ventilated patients.

Fentanyl is the drug of choice for continued pain management in these patients, regardless of hemodynamic status. That's right, despite their hemodynamic status. Fentanyl is very good on overall blood pressure and hemodynamic stability. When administering smaller aliquots, Fentanyl can be the perfect choice for hemodynamically unstable patients needing pain management in the mechanically ventilated setting. In my clinical experience, I have truly never had a patient decompensate more or drop their MAP because of my Fentanyl administration. Oftentimes, patients will benefit from as low as 50 to 100 mcg doses. However, we have to remember that the drug has a very quick half-life and will wear off. Because of this, give Fentanyl every 5-8 minutes to maintain a good therapeutic threshold.

Fentanyl is also a medication that will have secondary sedative effects when the overall total dose reaches 3-5mcg/kg. There have been many studies lately on the issue of delirium, from secondary benzodiazepine administration in the ICU dependent, mechanically ventilated patient. Based on those studies, many level 1 ICUs have gone away from the standard, historical benzodiazepine administration, and gone to Fentanyl drips to maintain both a level of pain management and sedation.

With that being said, Fentanyl use in the operating room with anesthesia for patient induction is looked at much different. With patients that have underlying heart disease and are being prepared for CABG, Anesthesiologist and CRNA's will use high dose Fentanyl for induction only. They don not use Etomidate, Ketamine, Propofol or paralytics like Succinylcholine, only high dose Fentanyl at huge doses. Standard dose will be 700-900 mcg per IVP over 2-3 minutes. This is for fragile hearts, with associated left ventricular dysfunction. I know that the operating room is not the pre-hospital environment and studies need to be conducted to ascertain the correlation between these two types of patient settings and how trauma patients, sepsis and other disease processes will handle higher dose fentanyl.

In the end, please be kind to your patients and administer Fentanyl in liberal dosing strategies. This is more important than your sedation with medications like Versed or Valium. Remember that despite an unstable patient, you still need to administer pain management. Fentanyl will not drop your pressure. Lastly, our pain response is sympathetic in nature. The sympathetic response associated will increase oxygen demand, metabolic rates, ICP and worsen any decompensation.

Ketamine
- **Non-barbiturate anesthetic**
    - Dose: 1-2 mg/kg IV – RSI Induction
        - 4mg/kg IV or IM – Excited Delirium
        - 0.1-0.25mg/kg IV – Pain Management
        - 0.5-0.1mg/kg IV - Sedation
    - Route: IV/IO

- **Onset: Variable**
- **Duration: Variable**
- **Indications: sedation for induction with severe bronchospasm, analgesia, ongoing sedation, excited delirium**
- **Contraindications: allergy to drug components, hypertension**

Ketamine - the wonder drug! That is how I refer to this amazing, but often very misunderstood medication. Ketamine has amazing properties that will enhance your ability to treat sick, hemodynamically unstable, mechanically ventilated patients. Ketamine is a medication that gives you the ability to treat sedation, with its anesthetic properties, as well as analgesia, by its excellent pain management properties.

I think there has been a major misconception formed about Ketamine and it is only based on fallacy. My experience with Ketamine has been truly amazing. It has surpassed my love for Fentanyl as my favorite medication. Obviously there are many reasons why Ketamine can be the drug of choice in our patient care. Most importantly is the application of treating sedation and pain in unstable, mechanically ventilated patients. The medication acts specifically on the thalamocortical and limbic systems, which control our sense, perception, emotion and memory. Because of this mechanism of action it works well by blocking our pain response.

Another big point to make about Ketamine that fits the treatment strategies related to hemodynamic compromise in our mechanically ventilated patients is its mechanism of action as a muscarinic receptor antagonist. Muscarinic receptors are said to be cholinergic in nature. So they provide a parasympathetic response. Based on the anticholinergic effects and positive central nervous system effects, the medication will actually cause an increase in blood pressure, mean arterial pressure and cardiac output. In the setting of hemodynamic compromise you can say that this response is very much welcomed. Lastly, the medication causes an increase in cerebral blood flow (CBF) by up to 60% and has an excellent effect on beta-2 receptors, causing bronchial dilation.

Ketamine does have a few side effects that need to be mentioned. The first one that comes to mind is the phenomenon of hypersalivation. This is very common in the pediatric population and something that you should expect. The treatment is administration of Atropine at 0.02mg/kg IVP. Suction often and continue to maintain a patent ETT until the Atropine takes effect. The second common side effect that many people worry about is the incidence of "emergence phenomenon". This actually happens <12% of the time, so in retrospect it is not as common as you would think. There has been many misconceptions regarding emergence phenomenon and more fallacy based assumptions, and nothing more. If you do have a patient that experiences this phenomenon, simple reassurance will help. Oftentimes reassurance prior to administering the medication will take care of any violent issues. However, if you do see this manifest, simply give a small dose of Versed or Valium and it will take care of the response.

Another issue you may encounter is laryngospasms. When giving Ketamine always administer the medication via IV push slowly, with the dose being pushed over 1 minute minimum. Giving Ketamine too rapidly will potentially cause laryngospasm, which can obviously be problematic with attempting airway management and intubation. If this does happen you can perform a technique called "Larson Maneuver". This is a technique where you perform a modified jaw thrust, but while doing this you place your middle fingers in the laryngospasm notches that lie anterior to the mastoid process of the temporal bone (essentially those little notches behind your ear lobe that your DAD used as a pressure point). Push bilaterally in a cephalad direction while performing a modified jaw thrust. This should reduce or stop the laryngospasm.

Lastly, countless research articles show its positive effects on our patient's response to the medication and dispel any arguments against Ketamine. One of those misconceptions is the argument of potential increases in ICP because of the increases seen in cerebral blood flow. However this has been shown to be without merit; with studies showing patients with traumatic brain injury having a reduction in ICP after Ketamine administration. In addition, consider what drives up ICP the most...it is pain. That is why we treat our patients with more liberal pain management strategies and use Fentanyl as our go to agent of choice. Couple that with correct Ketamine dosing strategies and you will have a patient that is very comfortable!

Versed
- **Benzodiazepine**
  - **Dose: 1-5mg**
  - **Route: IV/IO**
  - **Onset: 3-5 minutes**
  - **Duration: Variable (short-acting)**
  - **Indications: sedation for anxiety and ongoing sedation in mechanically ventilated patients**
  - **Contraindications: allergy to drug components and hypotension**

Versed is a potent, intermediate acting benzodiazepine that is used for sedation in the mechanically ventilated patient. Historically, the medication was used as the initial induction agent prior to your induction paralytic (Succinylcholine). In addition, the medication has been the go-to sedation medication for clinicians worldwide. It is actually really intriguing to think about the amount of Versed used on a daily basis and its potential negative side effects. When you compare this to Ketamine and all the fallacy involved with the medication, it is very comical to me. There have been thousands and thousands of documented deaths related to Versed, however in comparison very few with Ketamine. I would go all the way and say no directly related deaths with Ketamine, but I cannot verify that. My point is that we have accepted Versed in the industry for first line sedation despite its potential problems. However, it is a very dangerous drug with regards to respiratory depression and potential hemodynamic compromise.

Now that I have said my peace on Versed, we can now jump into the application aspects of the medication. Despite me tearing the medication down in the above paragraph, I still use Versed on all my patients and think it is an excellent medication if you use it correctly. Obviously I have my views on treatment and administration ranges, but feel like smaller doses are best. I tend to never go over 2.5 mg on continued sedation doses in mechanically ventilated patients. The old adage of: ***"You can't take it back, but can always give more"*** is very true with regards to Versed. In addition, many of our patients are hemodynamically unstable and you may see a reduction in blood pressure and mean arterial pressure with larger dosing strategies.

Versed still has its place in the critical care transport environment. I think if it is used correctly and consideration is taken for its potency and secondary effects on hemodynamics, you will see positive effects and will be pleased with how the medication performs. Lastly, protocols are going to drive your decision to use Versed or Ketamine. With that being said, if I had a choice, I would pick Ketamine over Versed 10 times out of 10.

Paralytics (Vecuronium and Rocuronium)

Vecuronium
- **Non-depolarizing neuromuscular blocking agent**
    - Dose: 0.1mg/kg
        - 0.01mg/kg for defasciculating dose

- Route: IV/IO
- Onset: 2 min
- Duration: 45-60 min
- Indications: long-term paralysis
- Contraindications: allergy to drug components, unsecured airway

Rocuronium
- Non-depolarizing neuromuscular blocking agent
  - Dose: 0.6-1.2 mg/kg
  - Route: IV/IO
  - Onset: 55-70 sec
  - Duration: 30-60 min
  - Indications: paralysis for induction and continuation
  - Contraindications: allergy to drug components

Maintaining good pain management and sedation as we have discussed above is one of the biggest aspects of maintaining a patient on the ventilator. Over the years we have seen many studies that have shown negative effects when using long-acting paralytics for intubated and mechanically ventilated patients. Gone are the days of giving a small dose of Versed and then dosing with Vecuronium or Rocuronium. I sure remember those days. With that being said...times have changed. Based on what we know about pain levels in intubated and mechanically ventilated patients, the focus now is all about pain management. One study showed that crews that gave long-acting paralysis forgot about the pain and sedation aspect and had periods between dosing of up to 30 minutes. The reason, they determined later, was because of the lack of movement from the patient. We have to remember however that just because they cannot move does not mean they cannot feel pain or are not aware of what is going on around them.

Furthermore, we now have excellent pain medications like Fentanyl and drugs like Ketamine that work well. One of the things I have tried to change in my approach to managing patients on the ventilator is how I deal with the long-acting paralysis issue. Once I realized that we as clinicians do not treat patients therapeutically with regards to pain and sedation when we give long-acting paralysis, I completely changed my approach and challenged myself to manage patients liberally, with Fentanyl specifically, but thoroughly with sedation as well. I can honestly say that I have not given Rocuronium or Vecuronium for long-acting paralysis for nearly four years now.

The shift in my approach is multi-layered. First, I am very liberal with continuous pain management with Fentanyl every 5 minutes. I also give Versed after every two doses of Fentanyl. Example: I will give one dose of Fentanyl at 100 mcg, then five minutes later will give another 100 mcg of Fentanyl as well as a dose of Versed at 2.5 mg. I continue to do this throughout the flight and will up my Fentanyl dose based on their weight and how they respond. I often remain with 2.5 mg doses of Versed for most patients. I also maintain patients on SIMV + PS and allow them small, triggered spontaneous breaths.

Obviously there may be those patients that are on chronic pain medications, benzodiazepines, or have ingested drugs like cocaine and meth that will change how they respond to the Fentanyl and Versed doses. In those cases it may be warranted to give Rocuronium or Vecuronium for safety purposes, however I think those examples are rare and we now have Ketamine that works great for those types of patients. I think most of the time for clinicians it is about "we've always done it this way", which is a product of culture. I also think it is about being lazy for some crews. They do not want to deal with a patient throughout the flight and give long-acting paralysis for that reason only. That is poor care and does not match the culture or example we should be setting as critical care providers.

Chapter 8 – Case Application Commentary

Case 1

Look at the ventilator settings and ABGs below and make the necessary ventilator changes.

ABGs: pH 6.96, PaCO$_2$ 18, HCO3- 13, PaO$_2$ 109, 80 kg
Current vent settings: SIMV 16, V$_t$ 500, f 38, FiO$_2$ 1.0, I:E 1:2, PIP 20, Pplat 16, PEEP 5
Labs: Na+ 138, Cl- 102, K+ 2.1, Glu 611

Patient was intubated for suspected DKA. Identify potential problems/treatment considerations.

Rationale:

The biggest aspect in regards to this patient presentation is the metabolic acidosis and DKA. Make sure you match the patient's spontaneous rate or match their EtCO$_2$ prior to intubation. Any change in PaCO$_2$ will affect pH in the opposite direction. A 10 mmHg increase will cause a decrease in 0.08 in pH. With a pH of 6.96, any changes in the patient's respiratory rate will be significant. Based on that, utilize the 240mL/kg/min calculation so as to maintain minute ventilation for proper pH protection. In addition, the K+ is 2.1 and is critically low. Any increase in pH of 0.10 will potentially cause a decrease in K+ by 0.6. As you can see, this patient

needs K⁺ administration as well, a 10-40 mEq run via IV and/or NGT administration, or by mouth. I would then run K⁺ at 10-20 mEq/hr for continued protection. It is always best to give the K⁺ because of the slow corresponding rise in serum K⁺ during infusion. For every 10 mEq given the corresponding rise is 0.1 in K⁺.

Case 2

Your aircraft is toned for an inter-facility transport from a small ICU back to the famous hospital "Rampart General". You arrive to find a 58-year-old, 60kg patient that has just been resuscitated from cardiac arrest after being intubated. The patient has a history of COPD, lung CA and upper GI bleed. The patient had presented to the ER earlier today with the complaint of "coughing up blood". She was transferred by local EMS to the hospital you are currently picking her up at. Once she arrived in the transferring ER, she started having respiratory distress that progressed rapidly to respiratory arrest. The ER physician elected to RSI and intubate. ETT placement was verified with BS. Successful intubation was performed after 2 attempts. Shortly after intubation the ER physician noted her to "brady" down and arrest. She was resuscitated via 5 minutes of CPR and 2 doses of Epi 1:10,000.

On arrival to the facility, you note the patient lying semi-fowler, intubated and on the mechanical ventilator. You note she is restless and having very fast, shallow respirations with very little chest rise. The transferring nurse states she has just got labs back and they are as follows:

VS: BP 98/52, P 105, SpO$_2$ 88%
ABGs: pH 6.97, PaCO$_2$ 17, HCO3- 10, PaO$_2$ 130
Current vent settings: AC 18, V$_t$ 650, f 34, PEEP 5, FiO$_2$ 0.40, PIP 83, P$_{plat}$ 58

What are your treatment options? What other information would you like?

Treatment Questions:

- *Obstructive or injury approach?*
- *Do you want protection with V$_t$ or RR?*
- *Why are the ABG results significant?*
- *What is causing the poor ventilation?*
- *How can we correct the high PIP and P$_{plat}$?*
- *How can we tell what the patient's auto-PEEP is?*
- *What changes to the current ventilator settings would benefit this patient?*

Rationale:

This is a very sick patient with multi-system failures. The first thing you should have identified and considered was the patient's cardiac arrest period. When did that happen? It happened shortly after intubation and was potentially due to a low pH. The patient's compensation was removed during the RSI process and the pH dropped because of the increase in PaCO$_2$ and corresponding related decrease in pH. Remember, for every change in PaCO$_2$ by 10 mmHg,

you will have an opposite change in pH by 0.08. During the intubation process, the $PaCO_2$ likely increased causing the corresponding drop in pH to critical lows, thus causing cardiac arrest.

Based on the patient's past medical history and current presentation I would consider the obstructive approach. I would immediately recommend assessing breath sounds and overall chest compliance. If this patient has little air movement, I would disconnect the ventilator and allow her to exhale. The poor compliance is associated with the underlying COPD history with air-trapping and auto-PEEP.

The next thing you should evaluate is the patient's current ventilator settings along with the assessment findings related to the poor chest rise and current PIP at 83 and P_{plat} at 58. These are critically high and need to be addressed immediately. I would first evaluate the pathophysiology and identify if I can correct something now. Second, the patient's V_t is 650 mL, and should be 360 mL based on her weight of 60 kg calculating at 6mL/kg. Re-evaluation of the P_{plat} would be my next goal. Most likely you will not see the P_{plat} reduce to <30 cmH_2O.

The patient is currently on AC-Vol, with her overbreathing the ventilator by 14 a minute. It would be better to switch her to SIMV, along with PCV so as to give her the best option to take spontaneous breaths, and to move her to a compliance-based mode of delivery. This will reduce anxiety and help with lowering the breath stacking and secondary air-trapping. With all that being said, remember the patient has a pH of 6.97. The obstructive approach is all about lowering the respiratory rate and optimizing exhalation. However, with a pH that low, the patient needs to be over-breathing the ventilator like she is and you will need to optimize the exhalation instead by affecting the I:E ratio. I would move the I:E ratio to 1:4.1 – 1:6.1 respectively.

I would then give the patient a small dose of pain medication. This is always a must with every patient on the ventilator. I would recommend starting with a small dose of 50mcg of Fentanyl and see if this allows you to optimize her ventilation.

If you recall our discussion on auto-PEEP and the application of external PEEP, we need to evaluate if the external PEEP is causing a problem. We accomplish this by evaluating the auto-PEEP and doing an expiratory hold. We never want to have the external PEEP 75-85% of the total auto-PEEP. Her current external PEEP is 5 cmH_2O, and based on that amount I would leave this alone for now.

The patient has a current SpO_2 of 88% on 40% FiO_2. I would increase my FiO_2 to 50% and re-evaluate the SpO_2. The goal is to slowly increase the FiO_2 until you hit >93% SpO_2. I would continue to evaluate my PIP and consider an in-line nebulizer during transport. I would also continue to administer Fentanyl and consider Ketamine for continued pain and sedation.

This will help as well with the COPD exacerbation with the bronchial dilation properties.

Case 3

You are dispatched for a scene flight, MVC with a 4-year-old male, 20kg, ejected approximately 16'.

The patient has obvious head trauma with a GCS of 8. You and your partner decide to perform RSI with successful intubation with a 5.0 ETT. You have a good $EtCO_2$ waveform present at 38 mmHg and bilateral BS are present.

Patient is placed on the ventilator – SIMV 22, V_t 120, PS 10, PEEP 5, PIP 28 cmH2O, P_{plat} 23 cmH2O. Approximately 10 minutes later you notice a sharp spike in your $EtCO_2$ and have a reading of 68 mmHg, PIP 42 cmH2O and P_{plat} 38 cmH2O.

Current V/S: BP 110/67, P 120, $EtCO_2$ 68

Treatment Questions:

- *Obstructive or injury approach?*
- *Do you want protection with V_t or RR?*
- *How can we correct the high PIP and P_{plat}?*
- *How can we tell what the patient's P_{plat} is?*
- *What is the primary treatment for this patient?*

Rationale:

Pediatric calls or flights can be stressful for any crew. You should have identified the ventilator strategy as the injury approach. Remember that any patient that does not fall under the COPD or asthma pathophysiology falls under the injury approach, even if they are intubated for something as simple as alcohol intoxication.

The big teaching point with this case is the primary and secondary assessment. If you are reading this from the perspective of a flight crewmember, you know that this assessment is pivotal. Once you load your patient into the aircraft, ongoing assessment with regards to chest trauma and any specific tension pneumothorax is limited to a few things. Any breath sound assessment on a pediatric patient's chest needs to be done at the most axillary point, due to the potential echoing heard from the opposite lung field. In addition, often times you will hear abdominal sounds and mistake those sounds for lung sounds, despite a pneumothorax.

The biggest red flag with the ventilator pressures are based on the initial P_{plat} of 23 cmH2O and then the follow up P_{plat} of 38 cmH2O. If you recall from our section on P_{plat}, we check this by doing a 0.5 sec inspiratory hold. If you see a change in P_{plat} >30 cmH2O, the first thing you should always think is that a tension pneumothorax is developing or has developed. Obviously other things can cause high P_{plat}, but with this patient's mechanism of injury, other injuries and the initial P_{plat} of 23 cmH2O, immediate chest decompression is warranted. If you have no idea which side is affected then do bilateral chest decompressions because this is considered life threatening.

You can also see that the blood pressure, pulse and SpO_2 have not changed. This is an important teaching point as well. Never wait for those things to change as these are late signs and indicate impending decompensation. In addition, tracheal deviation and poor BVM compliance are late signs as well and should never be clinical indicators for chest decompression procedures. Lastly, the $EtCO_2$ increase should immediately show you that there is a poor compliance issue and gas exchange is being hindered. This will show up earlier than chest wall compliance issues.

The main reason I wanted to discuss this case is due to the difficulty in assessing a pneumothorax and tension pneumothorax in intubated, mechanically ventilated patients. In addition, pediatric patients will compensate despite true clinical signs of impending collapse, with adult patients not showing clinical signs of hemodynamic changes in BP until they have 30-40% of their blood volume lost and pediatric having 25% loss respectively. This means not waiting for V/S changes in these patients. It is even more important to error on the side of caution and stay ahead of the game. I flew this patient and learned the hard way. I waited too long because of all the other clinical indicators that showed stable. However, the P$_{plat}$ is the most sensitive indicator of alveolar health. In the trauma setting and secondary mechanisms, any change seen above 30 cmH2O from baseline should be looked at as a tension pneumothorax and treated based on that parameter alone.

Case 4

You respond to a small tertiary hospital for a transfer out of the ICU. Initial report from the RN is a patient with COPD exacerbation that was intubated yesterday.

Current vent settings: SIMV 32, PC 30, V$_{te}$ 400, PEEP 15 cmH$_2$O, FiO$_2$ 1.0, SpO$_2$ of 88%, PIP 55, P$_{plat}$ 26

Current ABG results that were just drawn prior to your arrival show a pH 7.12, PaCO$_2$ 88, PaO$_2$ 235, and HCO3$^-$ 26

The RN also says that ABGs as of 1 hour ago showed pH 7.25, PaCO$_2$ 80 and PaO$_2$ 230

The RN advises you that they are unsure why the patient's ABG results are worse and they are now only getting a V$_{te}$ 210 mL based on the same PC 30

Treatment Questions:

- *Obstructive or injury approach?*
- *Do you want protection with V$_t$ or RR?*
- *Why are the ABG results worse?*

- What is causing the decrease in Vt and poor ventilation?
- What two ways can you use to identify the problem?
- How can you tell what the patient's auto-PEEP is?
- What changes to the current ventilator settings would benefit this patient?

Rationale:

This is that classic obstructive lung patient. Remember that your protection is all about allowing for exhalation and optimizing expiratory time by lowering the respiratory rate, lengthening the I:E ratio to 1:4.1 – 1:5.1 for starters. The true protective aspect of the obstructive approach is lowering and controlling the respiratory rate. Based on that, you should have identified that the patient has a current respiratory rate of 32. This is counter-productive for a patient that is suffering from ventilatory failure. I would first evaluate if this is a set rate, or a rate based on poor pain management and sedation. Regardless, this needs to get dropped by at least half. However, before you ever drop someone's rate or minute ventilation, always evaluate if this is a compensatory response. Are they over-breathing the ventilator to protect the pH and an underlying metabolic acidosis? Obviously this may hamper things a bit and change your approach. With this patient you can see that the metabolic disorder shows an uncompensated respiratory acidosis. There is not worry for any compensation due to the fact that the $PaCO_2$ is 88 and the $HCO3^-$ is within normal range.

The ABGs worsened due to the decrease in minute ventilation depicted by the decreasing V_{te}. This will cause the $PaCO_2$ to increase and thus drop the pH..

Your patient has a PIP of 50 cmH2O and P_{plat} is 26 cmH2O; both to be expected. The PEEP however is 15 cmH$_2$O, which is very high. Despite using PEEP to reduce the workload of breathing in these patients, I would reduce this immediately to 5 cmH$_2$O. Remember the section on auto-PEEP and the strategies for adding external PEEP in these patients. This may be something to think about after you fix the current issues. The concerning thing about this patient's current status is that her V_{te} has dropped from the initial reading of 400 mL to 210 mL. That indicates significant air-trapping and potentially dangerous auto-PEEP.

One way we can identify the current auto-PEEP status is to do an expiratory hold on the ventilator. This will give you some insight into the level of air-trapping and associated auto-PEEP. Obviously we know that it is significant and the prior respiratory rate of 32 was causing much of the problem. With that being said, seeing a drop in V_{te} of close to 200 mL is significant and needs to be addressed now! One of the first things I would do is disconnect the ventilator circuit and allow the patient 10-15 seconds to exhale. Some pulmonologists will actually apply gentle pressure on the chest to help with exhalation while the circuit is disconnected.

The SpO$_2$ being 88% is not really concerning to me. We need to remember that this patient is living close to that range chronically and is mostly a "right" shift on the oxyhemoglobin dissociation curve. That means that she is dumping all of her O$_2$ stores to the tissues. Her PaO$_2$ reflects this with readings of 235 and 230 respectively. Additionally, patients with COPD will often become what is called polycythemic. This is caused by an overproduction of erythropoietin and red blood cells. With added red blood cells comes added 2,3-DPG (the crow bars that allow off loading of oxygen from the hemoglobin). In addition, because of the high concentration of red blood cells and corresponding hemoglobin, the patient will seem hypoxic because not all of the hemoglobin will be filled with oxygen. Additionally, based on the reduced affinity related to hemoglobin's offloading of oxygen to the tissues, your patient's SpO$_2$ will be lower than normal, with an associated higher PaO$_2$.

Lastly, having the patient on SIMV + PS with PC is great. I would not change this and see this as the mode and delivery method that I would use on this patient. If you had PRVC available to you, it would be a great choice as well. This patient is suffering from poor compliance and PCV is a compliance-based mode. Dropping the respiratory rate, making sure I:E ratio is 1:4.1 – 1:5.1, and dropping the PEEP to 5 cmH$_2$O will turn this patient around in no time. Watch the V$_{te}$ and make sure this trends back up to the initial readings of 400 mL. In addition, continue with pharmacological intervention and manage the pain and sedation liberally, while allowing for patient rest.

Case 5

Look at the ventilator settings and ABGs below and identify any potential ventilator changes.

pH 7.37, $PaCO_2$ 50, $HCO3^-$ 23, PaO_2 51; 70kg male
SIMV 18, V_t 740, FiO_2 0.50, I:E 1:2, PIP 46, P_{plat} 44, PEEP 5 cmH_2O

Rationale:

First, we need to recognize that this patient is in a compensated respiratory acidosis, with the classification of respiratory failure. Note, the patient has a $PaCO_2$ 50 and a PaO_2 51 (Respiratory failure = $PaCO_2$ ≥50 and a PaO_2 ≤60). Continuing, volume always equals increased pressure. Look at the IBW and how high the V_t is. I would suggest decreasing Vt to 420-450mL and re-evaluate the PIP and P_{plat}. The P_{plat} is high most likely due to the high Vt. If you remember from our section on P_{plat}, the three steps you take to reduce the P_{plat} are to:

1. **Identify any potential pathophysiology that may be causing the issue. Example: tension pneumothorax, heavy patients lying supine etc.**
2. **Identify the V_t and reduce this in segments of 1mL/kg down to 4mL/kg.**
3. **Switch to pressure control ventilation**

The respiratory rate and I: E ratios are appropriate. The PIP will most likely decrease once the P_{plat} decreases. Remember the PIP will always be the highest pressure and will increase if the P_{plat} increases.

Reference Charts
Oxygen Quick Reference Equations

Oxygen adjustment calculation	• $(FiO_2 \times P1)/P2$ • $P1$ = Barometric pressure at patient pickup location • $P2$ = Barometric pressure at flying altitude ***Important for PDA dependent neonates***
Measuring oxygen delivery	• $CaO_2 = [1.34 \times Hgb \times (SaO_2)] + PaO_2 \times 0.003$ ○ $CaO_2 \times Q = DO_2$ • DO_2 = Amount of oxygen delivered each minute • CaO_2 = Content of O_2 in the arteries
Measuring cellular uptake of oxygen	• Fick Formula = Cellular uptake of O_2 • $CvO_2 = [1.34 \times Hgb \times (SvO_2)] + PaO_2 \times 0.003$ • O_2ER = (Oxygen Extraction ratio) • $O_2ER = (CaO_2 - CvO_2) / CaO_2$ • Normal O_2ER is 25%.. Meaning that Hgb passing through lungs to be oxygenated are 75% saturated during homeostasis

PO_2	Atmospheric Concentration
PaO_2	Arterial Concentration
PAO_2	Alveolar Concentration

Desired VE Formula
(Accounts for dead space)

Standard hemostasis VE	60mL/kg/min
Intubated patient demand	100mL/kg/min
Intubated - metabolic acidosis demand	240mL/kg/min or match pre-intubation $EtCO_2$

Ventilator Quick Chart

Abbreviations	Term	Definitions
PIP	Peak inspiratory pressure	*Point of maximal airway pressure*
PEEP	Positive end-expiratory pressure	*Pressure maintained in airways at end of exhalation*
ΔP	Delta pressure	*Difference between PIP-PEEP / Driving Pressure*
V_t	Tidal volume	*Volume of gas entering patient's lungs during inspiration*
I_t	Inspiratory time	*The duration of time in inspiration*
E_t	Expiratory time	*The duration of time in expiration*
MAP	Mean airway pressure	*An average of the airway pressure throughout the respiratory cycle*
RR	Rate	*Respiratory rate as set on the ventilator*

P_{plat}	Plateau pressure	*Amount of pressure placed against alveoli showing alveolar health*
FiO₂	Fraction of inspired oxygen	*Percentage of oxygen from 0.21 – 1.0*
I:E ratio	Inspiratory vs. expiratory time	*The ratio of the duration of inspiration to the duration of expiration time*
Pinsp	Inspiratory pressure	*Inspiratory pressure for pressure initiated ventilation*
PS	Pressure support	*Pressure applied at the end of vent circuit; used in SIMV to augment the patient's spontaneous breath*
C_{stat}	Static compliance = $C_{stat} = \dfrac{V_T}{P_{plat} - PEEP}$	*Compliance during periods without gas flow, such as during an inspiratory pause*

I-Time – I:E ratio chart

Respiratory Rate	I-Time	I:E ratio
10	2.0	1:2
12	1.5	1:2.3
15	1.3	1:2.1
20	1.0	1:2.0
25	.8	1:2.0
30	.6	1:2.3

FlightBridgeED, LLC provides continuing education and advanced certification review courses that focus on FP-C, CCP-C, CFRN, CTRN, CCRN, and CEN review content and test preparation for nurses and paramedics, as well as other seminars on critical care topics. We offer these courses via live and on-demand delivery. It is our goal to consistently improve these courses and to provide the highest quality products that make you, the student, successful in your testing process and most importantly, your patient care!

We also offer FP-C, CCP-C or CFRN practice exams via our on-line learning management system. We offer this in package format with all review classes or as individual purchase options. You can purchase 1-week, 2-week and 4-week subscriptions, with unlimited attempts during that time period (visit www.flightbridgeed.com). These exams simulate the computer-based testing you will utilize during the actual certification exams.

You can also access free critical care education via our podcast series. You can find these on our website under the **"Blog"** category as well as via iTunes on your iPhone or via Google play on your android phone by searching **"The FlightBridgeED Podcast"**. In addition, check out the **"Second Shift Podcast"**. You can download the free podcast app and subscribe for automatic downloads bi-weekly via your iPhone or Android.

Would you like to host a live review course? Do you need ventilator training? We provide the only pre-hospital 1-day critical care focused ventilator workshop. Are you in need of other critical care continuing education? Contact us for course setup.
Contact: eric.bauer@flightbridgeed.com

We would love to hear your feedback and we'd appreciate you taking the time to let us know how we are doing and what we can do to serve you better.

Customer and instructional support:
eric.bauer@flightbridgeed.com
Tech Support: techsupport@flightbridgeed.com
Website: www.flightbridgeed.com

We appreciate your support and for allowing us to invest in your education!

References

American Association of Critical-Care Nurses. (2010). AACN practice alerts: Oral care for patients at risk for ventilator associated pneumonia. Retrieved from http://www.aacn.org/WD/Practice/Docs

ARDS Network. (1998). *Prospective, randomized, multi-center trial of 12 ml/kg vs. 6 ml/kg tidal volume positive pressure ventilation for treatment of acute lung injury and acute respiratory distress syndrome (ARMA).* ARDSNet Study 01, Version III. Retrieved from http://www.ardsnet.org/system/files/armaprotocolV3_1998-09-11_0.pdf

Brochard L, Harf A, Lorino H, Lemaire F. Inspiratory pressure support prevents diaphragmatic fatigue during weaning from mechanical ventilation. Am Rev Respir Dis. 1989;139:513-521.

Brochard, L, Rua F, Lorino H, Lemaire M, Harf A. Inspiratory pressure support compensates for the additional work of breathing caused by the endotracheal tube. Anesthesiology. 1991;75:739-745.

Cabodevila-Mireles, Eduardo, Kacmarek M, Robert. Should Airway Pressure Release Ventilation Be the Primary Mode in ARDS? Respiratory Care 2016;6(61):761-773

Charles. Ventilator-associated pneumonia. Australas Med J 2014;;7(8):334-44 http://dx.doi.org/10.4066/AMJ.2014.2105

Davies, RRT, J., Senussi, MD, M., & Cabodevila, MD, E. M. (2016, June 2016). Should A Tidal Volume of 6 mL/kg Be Used in All Patients? [Journal]. *Respiratory Care, 61*(6), 774-790.

DeLuca et al. (2013). Implementing a ventilator-associated pneumonia bundle in academic emergency department.
Eur J Emerg Med. 2013 Feb;20(1):61-3

Goldenberg. Lung-protective Ventilation in the Operating Room: Time to Implement? Anaesthesiology 2014;121;184-188
http://dx.doi.org/10.1097/ALN.0000000000000274

Klouwenberg. The attributable mortality of delirium in critically ill patients: prospective cohort study. BMJ 2014;349:g6652
http://dx.doi.org/10.1136/bmj.g6652

Kopman. Is Postoperative Residual Neuromuscular Block Associated with Adverse Clinical Outcomes? What Is the Evidence? Current Anesthesiology Reports 2013;3(2):114-121
http://dx.doi.org/10.1007/s40140-013-0009-6

McIntosh, L. (1997). *Essentials of nurse anesthesia.* New York: McGraw-Hill Companies Inc.

McCoy, T., Fields, W., Kent, N. (2011). Evaluation of Emergency Department Evidence –based practices to prevent the incidence of ventilator acquired pneumonia. Journal of Care Quality. Vol, No.1 pp83-88

Mughal, M. M., Minai, O., Culver, D., & Arroliga, A. (2005). Auto-positive end-expiratory pressure-Mechanisms and treatment. *Cleveland Clinical Journal Of Medicine*.

Neligan, P. (2006). Acute Lung Injury. Retrieved from Critical Care Medicine Tutorials: http://www.ccm tutorials.com/rs/ali/vili.htm

Rock. Sedation and Its Association With Posttraumatic Stress Disorder After Intensive Care. Crit Care Nurse 2014;34(1):30-37
http://dx.doi.org/10.4037/ccn2014209

Sleigh. Ketamine – More mechanisms of action than just NMDA blockade. Trends in Anaesthesia and Critical Care 2014;4(2):76-81
http://dx.doi.org/10.1016/j.tacc.2014.03.002

Tobin M, ed. *Pressure Support Ventilation in Principles and Practice of Mechanical Ventilation*. New York: McGraw-Hill, Inc; 1994:239-257.

Walls, R., Murphy, M., Luten, R., & Schneider, R. (2008). *The manual of emergency airway management*. (3rd Ed.). Philadelphia, PA: Lippincott Williams & Wilkin

Made in the USA
Columbia, SC
11 May 2019